Rowena 99

Overeaters Anonymous

Second Edition

Overeaters Anonymous®, Inc.
Rio Rancho, New Mexico USA

Overeaters Anonymous, Inc.

PO Box 44020, Rio Rancho NM 87174-4020 USA

505-891-2664

www.oa.org

© 1980, 2001 by Overeaters Anonymous, Inc.

Second Edition 2001.

Fifth Printing

Printed in the United States of America.

Library of Congress Catalog Card No.: 00-93501

ISBN: 1-889681-02-4

Contents

Contents

Foreword

I have had both a personal and professional interest in obesity for a great many years. The fact is I've been an overeater all of my life and a fat man most of my life. I did not understand the destructive aspects of overeating, however, until I began to practice psychiatry.

Eventually it became apparent to me that overeating is an obsessive, compulsive addiction of a highly complex nature. I became aware that food can be even more addictive than tobacco, drugs, alcohol, or gambling, and at least as destructive. The simple fact is that we cannot do without food, and each time the food addict eats he or she is in danger of succumbing to the compulsion.

The further facts are: (1) Food is usually available in abundance. (2) There is no societal, legal dictum against eating. (3) In many places overeating is encouraged. (4) Confusion about this highly complex syndrome abounds.

Indeed, there is still a great deal we do not know about overeating. But we do know now that one's emotional life has a great deal to do with overeating. I believe that repressed anger plays a powerful role in this addiction. I feel that eating binges are often displaced temper tantrums or rage reactions. I also believe that the roots of the condition can often be traced to the earliest times in our lives and to early and complicated family relations. Those who suffer from the problem and those who seriously engage in working in the area also know how malignant the condition is. This destructive aspect occurs relative to the victim's physical health, emotional well being, social life, professional life, sex life, and economic life.

We also know, unfortunately, how limited all treatment modalities have been to date in effecting sustained relief, let alone "cures." We know, too, how obese people have been patronized, prejudiced against, and exploited for economic gain. Charlatans and chicanery abound. Millions of dollars are made off the suffering of fat people, and this condition is probably the most prevalent health problem which exists in the American population. Of course, as with all other problems, there are varying degrees of difficulty and suffering. But the numbers of people who are driven to seek help make commercial enterprise in this field big business.

Overeaters Anonymous is not a business. This organization represents one of our country's major and perhaps largest efforts at self-help—real and effective self-help. OA enjoys a reputation for significant success in a field strewn with failure. OA's success goes beyond weight reduction and control, though this alone is an achievement of great magnitude. OA also helps to contribute a greater sense of self and self-esteem through its extraordinary implementation of camaraderie and caring for one's fellows and one's self. It functions as a giant contributor to awakening and adding to its members' sense of their own humanity. This is crucial in battling malignant addiction or, for that matter, any illness of the mind and body; they really are one.

This book describes the OA experience as told by various members through their own stories. These are moving and educational stories. They are full of struggle—constructive struggle—and hope. Most important, they tell of enhanced compassion for self, for others, and for the state of being human. They tell us about fellowship and what a powerful therapeutic instrument caring can be. They also tell us what

caring is all about. Read them and enjoy being part of the
human condition.

Theodore Isaac Rubin, M.D.

*Dr. Rubin is a well-known psychoanalyst practicing
psychiatry in New York City. He is past-president of the
American Institute for Psychoanalysis and has served on
many local and national medical boards. He is the author
of more than thirty books, translated worldwide, including*
Compassion and Self-Hate, Lisa and David, Jordi, The
Winner's Notebook, *and* Lisa and David Today. *Among
the many honors he has won are the Adolph Meyer Award
from the Association for the Improvement of Mental Health
and the Social Conscience Award from the Karen Horney
Clinic, a psychiatric institution.*

Acknowledgement _____

This book would not be possible without our great preceptor, Alcoholics Anonymous. Indeed, many of those whose contributions appear in these pages would not be among us today without the Steps and Traditions of the AA program.

In publishing this collection of personal stories of recovery, Overeaters Anonymous has only one purpose: to describe for all who may be interested the progression of our illness, what we found in this program and how it has changed us. Our book is not intended as a substitute for or a replacement of Alcoholics Anonymous, the life-giving "Big Book" which has brought physical, emotional, and spiritual rebirth to millions around the globe.

Those of us who speak in these pages confirm the prophetic words used in 1951 in conferring the Lasker Award on the then sixteen-year-old Fellowship of Alcoholics Anonymous:

". . . Historians may one day recognize Alcoholics Anonymous to have been a great venture in social pioneering which forged a new instrument for social action; a new therapy based on the kinship of common suffering; one having a vast potential for the myriad other ills of mankind."

Our deepest gratitude to the Fellowship of Alcoholics Anonymous for their continued growth without promotion, exemplary leadership without leaders, and principles without personalities.

*QA*___

Our Invitation to You

WE OF OVEREATERS ANONYMOUS have made a discovery. At the very first meeting we attended, we learned that we were in the clutches of a dangerous illness, and that will power, emotional health, and self-confidence, which some of us had once possessed, were no defense against it.

To be sure, the picture painted of the disease was grim: progressive, debilitating, incurable. Compulsive overeating has many symptoms in addition to mere fat. It is also an illness which isolates and gradually, or rapidly, causes increasingly serious problems in one or more areas of our lives: health, job, finances, family, or social life.

No one is sure what causes it; probably a number of factors: environment, a certain way of reacting to life, biological predisposition.

We have learned that the reasons are unimportant. What deserves the attention of the still-suffering compulsive overeater is this: *there is a proven, workable method by which we can arrest our illness.*

The OA recovery program is patterned after that of Alcoholics Anonymous. We use AA's Twelve Steps and Twelve Traditions, changing only the words "alcohol" and "alcoholic" to "food" and "compulsive overeater."

As the personal stories in this book attest, the Twelve-Step program of recovery works as well for compulsive overeaters as it does for alcoholics. Our members prove that compulsive overeaters can share their problems and help each other, thus benefiting not only themselves but their families and the communities in which they live.

Can we guarantee *you* this recovery? The answer is simple. If you will honestly face the truth about yourself and the illness; if you will keep coming back to meetings to talk and listen to other recovering compulsive overeaters; if you will read our literature and that of Alcoholics Anonymous with an open mind; and, most important, if you are willing to rely on a power greater than yourself for direction in your life, and to take the Twelve Steps to the best of your ability, we believe you can indeed join the ranks of those who recover.

The disease of compulsive overeating causes or contributes to illness on three levels—emotional, physical, and spiritual. To remedy this threefold illness we offer several suggestions, but the reader should keep in mind that the basis of the program is spiritual, as evidenced by the Twelve Steps.

We are not a "diet and calories" club. We do not endorse any particular plan of eating. We practice abstinence by staying away from eating between planned meals and from all individual binge foods. Once we become abstinent, the preoccupation with food diminishes and in many cases leaves us entirely. We then find that, to deal with our inner turmoil, we have to have a new way of thinking, of acting on life rather than reacting to it—in essence, a new way of living.

From this vantage point, we begin the Twelve-Step program of recovery, moving beyond the food and the emotional havoc to a fuller living experience.

We believe that no amount of will power or self-determination could have saved us. Times without number, our resolutions and plans were shattered as we saw our individual resources fail.

So we honestly admitted to ourselves that we were powerless over food. This was the first step toward recovery. It followed that, if we had no power of our own, we needed a power outside ourselves to help us recover.

Some of us, including agnostics and atheists, regard the group itself as a power greater than ourselves. Others choose to accept different interpretations of this power. But most of us adopt the concept of God as God may be understood by each individual.

As a result of practicing the Steps, the symptom of compulsive overeating is removed on a daily basis. Thus, for most of us, abstinence means freedom from the bondage of compulsive overeating, achieved through the process of surrendering to something greater than ourselves; the more total our surrender, the more fully realized our freedom from food obsession.

Here are the Steps as adapted for Overeaters Anonymous:

1. We admitted we were powerless over food—that our lives had become unmanageable.

2. Came to believe that a Power greater than ourselves could restore us to sanity.

3. Made a decision to turn our will and our lives over to the care of God *as we understood Him*.

4. Made a searching and fearless moral inventory of ourselves.

5. Admitted to God, to ourselves, and to another human being the exact nature of our wrongs.

6. Were entirely ready to have God remove all these defects of character.

7. Humbly asked Him to remove our shortcomings.

8. Made a list of all persons we had harmed and became willing to make amends to them all.

9. Made direct amends to such people wherever possible, except when to do so would injure them or others.

10. Continued to take personal inventory, and when we were wrong, promptly admitted it.

11. Sought through prayer and meditation to improve our conscious contact with God *as we understood Him*, praying only for knowledge of His will for us and the power to carry that out.

12. Having had a spiritual awakening as the result of these Steps, we tried to carry this message to compulsive overeaters and to practice these principles in all our affairs.*

"How can I face this?" you may ask. We suggest you do so only one day at a time. "Just for today" is one of many deeply meaningful OA slogans. "I can do anything for twenty-four hours that I couldn't do for a lifetime" was a brand new way of thinking for us. Before, we looked at our weight problem—and all our other problems—and said, "What's the use? It's too much for me. I can't possibly do it."

---

*Reprinted by permission of AA World Services, Inc.

Now, we fully accept and live by the premise that we don't have to look at everything all at once. We know that it's necessary to do a certain amount of planning but, once having planned, we act for this one day alone.

"But I'm too weak. I'll never make it!" Don't worry; we have all thought and said the same thing. The amazing secret to the success of this program is just that: weakness. It is weakness, not strength, that binds us to each other and to a higher power and somehow gives us an ability to do what we cannot do alone. We have discovered that if people in this program love us, it is not for our strength, but for our weakness and our willingness to share that with others.

After reading the personal stories in this book, you may proclaim, "I'm not *that* bad!" Once again, we ask you to keep in mind that compulsive overeating is a progressive illness. If you really are a compulsive overeater, the symptoms will grow worse. Within our ranks are those who were recovering but tried once again to control food by their own devices, with consequent return to serious overeating and, in many cases, massive weight gain.

If you can identify with the developing pattern of overeating revealed in our stories, you probably are a compulsive overeater. The chances are that your symptoms will eventually reach those of late-stage compulsive overeating. In other words, you're not that bad—yet!

If, after reading this book, you decide you are one of us, we welcome you with open arms. You are not alone any more! Overeaters Anonymous extends to all of you the gift of acceptance. No matter who you are, where you come from or where you are going, you are welcome here. Regardless of what you have done or failed to do, what you have felt or haven't felt, who you have loved or hated, you may be sure of our unconditional acceptance.

We will help you and rejoice with you and tell you that we are not failures just because we sometimes fail. We'll hold out our arms in love and stand beside you as you pull yourself back up and walk on again to where you are heading.

Sometimes *we* fail to be all that we could be, and sometimes we aren't there to give you all you need from us. Accept our imperfections, too. Love and help us in return. That is what we are in OA—imperfect but progressing. Let us rejoice together in our recovery and in the assurance that we have a home, if we want it.

Welcome to Overeaters Anonymous. Welcome home!

1

Keep Coming Back: Rozanne's Story

"HONEY, IF YOU HAVE a twenty-three-inch waist, everything else will be all right." My mother's words were to haunt me all my growing-up years. The promise that a slender figure would bring instant and permanent happiness was an illusion in which I believed with all my heart. The few times I was thin, nothing else changed. I thought that the fault was mine. "If only I tried harder," I told myself, "everything would be different." The persistence of my illusion was astonishing.

Trying harder was our family tradition. I come from a family of superachievers and compulsive overeaters. My mother grew up in Green Bay, Wisconsin, in the early 1900's. In that small town my grandfather owned the first movie theaters and the first automobile. My grandmother was very daring for those times—she supported Margaret Sanger several years before Sanger founded Planned Parenthood. My father was world famous in his own right in B'nai B'rith, an international Jewish organization. My mother was one of America's first dieticians in the early 1920s.

My parents were loving perfectionists, and both were extremely education oriented. My younger brother and I learned early that the way to be worth anything was to work very hard and to achieve beyond the scope of most other people. Growing up, we believed that just being a loving person wasn't enough; we had to excel to be worthwhile.

In my very early teens, I decided I wanted to be a famous actress, pretending to be someone else, noticed and applauded for my efforts and talent. Maybe then I would be acceptable.

Born in Milwaukee, Wisconsin, I moved with my family to Chicago when I was twelve. Sadly, I'd been an overweight child, and now I was becoming a very pudgy teenager. Often I heard well-meaning people say, "You have such a pretty face, dear. If only you'd lose weight." That broke my heart. Did it mean I wasn't any good because I was fat? I just tried a little harder, worked a little more, studied a little longer.

None of it had any effect. You see, buried in my soul was the secret I told no one—I hated myself—and no amount of superachieving could bring me peace of mind.

As I entered my third year at the University of Chicago, I had just turned eighteen. It seemed that all the other girls were dating, but I was alone in my dorm room on Saturday nights. It was obvious that being fat would never attract boys, so I made a decision to give up overeating. At 142 pounds, I went on a diet, and for the first time in my life I became thin. I was five-feet-two-inches and weighed 118 pounds.

Suddenly the boys began to notice me. I had so many

dates, I began to neglect my studies and flunked every subject. I can still feel my parents' anger and disappointment. My furious father insisted on sending me to business school. "Not only will you learn your lesson," he said, "but you'll gain some skills with which to earn a living." (It was this excellent training which prepared me for setting up the first OA office in my dining room ten years later.) Unfortunately, I returned to overeating and regained all the weight I had lost. The following year I returned to put myself through the University and earn a BA degree.

After graduation, I began working as a producer's secretary in a local summer theater. There I met Imogene Coca, a famous television comedienne. I told her I was going to New York City in the fall to find work in the theater or television. "Be sure to call me," she urged, "and I'll help you find a job." My famous friend kept her word, and I soon found myself working as a producer's secretary at NBC on TV specials with Bob Hope, Eddie Cantor, and Kate Smith.

In that position, I could see the constant rejections received by auditioning actors and actresses. My own fear of rejection was so strong that it overrode my lifelong acting ambition. I settled for working behind the scenes as a producer's secretary, where it was safe.

Those were the early days of commercial television, an exciting life for a young woman. Still I had no peace of mind. At 142 pounds I hated my body, but I couldn't seem to stop overeating.

In addition, I had developed a fierce resentment toward my mother and now blamed her for my unhappiness. (Years later, after much Twelve-Step work on myself, that resentment was removed, and I finally took responsibility for my own actions.)

After two years I returned home to Chicago, where I became a fashion copywriter at a large department store. At last I had found my lifelong vocational love: writing.

But youth is restless. My mother's mother lived in sunny Los Angeles, and I sensed an opportunity. "I've had enough of winter snow," I told my mother. "I'm going to California to live with Grandma and to find fame, fortune and a husband." In Los Angeles I again went to great lengths to find a boyfriend—I gave up excess food and became slender once more. After another copywriting stint, I became assistant advertising manager of a prestigious chain of department stores. The job was terrific, I was thin, men were calling me for dates, and life really seemed to be going my way.

Yet something was terribly wrong. What was it? No matter what happened, no matter how tiny I was, self-hate still ate at my very soul. I couldn't even admit it to myself.

In January 1955, I joined my girlfriend at a Sunday afternoon charity dance at the famous Ambassador Hotel. "Oh, look," said my friend, pointing across the room. "There's Marv S____. I dated him once. Come on, I'll introduce you."

After exchanging names, I looked up into the kindest eyes I'd ever seen. Smiling down at me was Marvin, my gentle, caring partner-to-be. I was twenty-six years old, I weighed 118 pounds, I was falling in love. Despite such wonders, I was barely hanging onto my diet. Old feelings still raged underneath, and old habits were biding their time, waiting for the crack in my armor.

Marvin proposed to me in August, and at our wedding four months later, I weighed 129 pounds. All it took was that little ring on my finger for me to take back the food.

That was only the beginning. Ten months later Debbie was born, and Julie came along seventeen months after that. By this time, life was too much for me. I weighed 148 pounds, with more fat piling on every day. I couldn't stop eating, and most of the time I wished I were dead. My self-worth was completely gone, my soul was empty, I had no place to go, and I didn't believe in God. What was left for me?

The answer came late one quiet November night in 1958. Marvin and my babies were asleep, and it was time for my usual routine of TV watching and eating. Twenty-nine years old and 152 pounds, I spent every night until bedtime filling my inner emptiness with excess food.

Paul Coates, a syndicated television journalist, hosted a weekly show called Paul Coates' Confidential File. That night he was interviewing a member from a new organization called Gamblers Anonymous. My husband had a friend who was a compulsive gambler, and I thought this might be just the thing for him. So Marvin and I took his friend to a GA meeting just before Thanksgiving.

As long as I live, I will never forget that night. We were in a meeting hall with about twenty-five men and a sprinkling of wives. Each man in turn got up and talked about his life of lying and cheating, stealing and hiding. Sitting in the back of that room with my big, black coat clutched around me, I was absolutely transfixed. "I'm just like that," I said to myself. "Their compulsion is with gambling and mine is with food, but now I know I'm not alone anymore!" I discovered that I wasn't wicked or sinful; I was sick. I had an illness, and I could give it a name—compulsive overeating. It was a revelation, and when I walked out of the meeting room that night, my life changed forever.

I wanted to talk to other overeaters, but I couldn't find any groups for people like me. Terrified, I didn't know where to turn. Years of conventional therapy had not helped my compulsive overeating. Where could I go? What should I do? Clinging to a diet for the next three weeks, I finally gave in and went back to my old ways. Helpless and hopeless, I didn't know that I needed other people for support and a life-changing program for recovery.

I continued to overeat and cry for another year. In November 1959, new neighbors moved in down the block. The woman, Jo S., weighed over two hundred pounds, and I'd never seen anyone who looked like her. When I saw her, I said to myself, "I'll never look like that. I'll never let myself weigh that much." Aren't those famous last words for an overeater?

Now, approaching a new year, I was only thirty years old, and I was fatter than I'd ever been. During the holidays, I had gained nine pounds in a week and a half! Now weighing 161 pounds, I wore a size twenty. I'd never weighed that much, never been that fat. Yet that was the catalyst that propelled me into action.

Despairing and desperate, I remembered that night at Gamblers Anonymous. I told my husband, "Marvin, I can't find any group, so I'm going back to Gamblers Anonymous to see if it's the same as I remember."

By late 1959 GA was two and a half years old; several of the men I'd heard before were still there, and they welcomed me warmly.

After the meeting, I approached Jim W., the founder of Gamblers Anonymous. It must have been quite a sight—a five-foot-two-inch, overweight young woman staring up into the face of a six-foot-two-inch, skinny, middle-aged man.

Heart pounding, I asked, "Jim, do you think an organization like yours could work for compulsive overeaters like me?" He smiled down at me gently. "I don't see why not. I was in Alcoholics Anonymous before I started GA."

There it was—a hand outstretched to steady me as I stumbled along. It was my first experience with the Twelfth Step, the first time anyone had offered to help me with no thought of reward. I went home and told Marvin, "I think I finally have a chance."

From the moment the idea occurred to me, I envisioned a Fellowship as big as AA or bigger, with meetings all around the world. "If the alcoholic is a compulsive overdrinker," I mused to myself, "then we must be compulsive overeaters. I'll call our organization Overeaters Anonymous."

Meanwhile, Christmas came and went. One crisp December afternoon I was strolling my babies down the block when I spied my overweight neighbor wheeling her baby across the street. "Here's my chance," I said to myself. "It's now or never!"

I joined her, and we chatted for a few minutes. As we approached my house, I blurted out, "Jo, I've got to rush. I have to go to the health club to see about starting this group."

"This group? What group?" she asked. "Well," I answered, "I know you don't share this problem, but I'm a compulsive overeater, and I'm having a terrible time."

Intrigued, she persisted. "What's the name of your group?"

I took a deep breath. "Overeaters Anonymous."

"You know," she offered, "I would be interested. I think I'd like to try it with you." At that moment, the Fellowship of Overeaters Anonymous was born.

I was elated and filled with hope. "Maybe I'll have a chance now," I said to myself. "I won't be alone anymore."

A few days later, during a physical checkup, my doctor said, "Rozanne, you need to lose about fifty pounds. I have just the pill to help you lose weight." Remember, this was the beginning of the 1960s. Along with many others, I was naive regarding drugs, and I viewed my doctor as The Authority. Overstimulated as a result of the medicine, I stopped excessive eating, and for six months I had the cleanest house in Los Angeles! During that period, I went from 161 pounds to 120 pounds and eventually to 110 pounds, a weight I maintained for several years. However, despite my dramatic weight loss, my heart and soul were still buried in self-hate, and I didn't know how to rescue myself. The medicine helped for the six months I took it, but my efforts to start OA were to be the most important factor in changing both my body and my inner sense of self-esteem.

In addition to my first two visits to GA, Jo had accompanied me to one more meeting. Neither of us knew anything about AA. On January 19, 1960, we held the first OA meeting. Jo and I were there, along with Bernice, the wife of a GA member. For all of us, it was a relief to be able to talk about our struggles with someone who understood.

Suddenly, during the start of the third meeting, Bernice said, "My doctor says dieting makes me nervous." With that she got up and walked out the door. Jo and I looked at each other. I was stunned and frightened. Was it over before it had started? Had I lost my only hope? Jo wanted to leave, but I started to cry and said that I couldn't do it alone, insisting that she had to stay. She agreed.

We struggled along. By August we had both lost a lot of

weight. Jo went from 200 pounds to 109 in nine months; I came down from 161 to 118 in the same time. Physically, we were splendid examples to prospective members.

However, in the beginning, the less I ate the more my anxieties and feelings of worthlessness rose to the surface. Because I couldn't admit them, even to myself, I covered everything with a lot of self-willed actions.

The first thing I decided was that those AA Steps were very poorly written. "That Bill W. (AA's cofounder) was only a stockbroker," I snickered to myself, "and I'm a professional writer. I can do a better job on the Steps." I thought I knew everything.

In addition, the training in my Jewish home had been more traditionally ethnic than spiritual. I believed that I was not so weak that I had to turn my life and my will over to the care of any God, whether He existed or not. Therefore, I removed AA's Step Three and wrote a new one.

Because I felt strongly about the importance of nutrition and calorie-counting, my new Step Three advocated consultation "with a physician of our own choosing." Adamant and defiant, I proceeded to remove the word "God" and all mention of spiritual concepts from the rest of the Steps. Then I took a good look at what I had done and realized that the Steps didn't look at all like those of AA.

"After all," I sighed, "I do want people to say we are like AA." So I reluctantly sprinkled God back into a few of the Steps. Neither Jo nor I knew any better.

OA became an integral part of my life from its beginning. I was obsessed with my vision, living and breathing it as I continued to care for my home and family. Most important, I had finally found someone to talk to, someone who understood my struggles with food.

After a few weeks I read my rewritten Steps to Jim W. He must have been horrified, but he'd talked to me enough to realize I was one of those examples of self-will run riot the AA "Big Book" talks about. I was starting my own game and making my own rules as I went along. Biding his time, he said nothing.

In April Barbara S. joined our little group. Now there were Jo and Barbara and me. Drifting in and out were several friends of ours. Nobody in our new little group had been to AA. I had been to three GA meetings; Jo had been to one GA meeting with me. During our weekly OA meetings we discussed our feelings on a psychological level. We knew nothing of the meaning of inventories or amends, and I bristled at the thought of surrender and spiritual awakening.

After a few weeks Jim suggested that we visit an AA meeting. "Oh, I couldn't," I shot back. "They might be drunk and accost us." Oh, the patience of Jim!

"No, no," he laughed, "the drunks are in many other places, but the sober ones are in the AA meetings." Trembling inside and very fearful, Jo and I went to an AA meeting.

That was an eye-opening experience for me. I listened to concepts I'd never heard before, and I felt a tangible love in the room. Unfortunately, my fears were in the way, and I was still unable to accept many of the basic precepts of the AA program, especially those contained in the original Twelve Steps. Most important, I refused to embrace the idea of surrendering my life and will to the care of a Higher Power.

The thinner I became and the more I achieved, the worse I felt. I didn't dare let people know this. They might find out how terrible I was. (I remember receiving a standing ovation when I was introduced at our first Conference in 1962. Later I confessed to my sponsor, Thelma, "If they knew how rotten I am, they wouldn't stand up and applaud, they would stand up and turn around and walk out!")

Jo left California and OA in August 1960. That left Barbara and me and five other women who resisted the OA program at every meeting. I was frightened. What would happen to my magnificent dream? By that time I weighed 117 pounds, and Barbara had gone down from 192 to 132 pounds. Physically, we were both programs of attraction. Finally, Paul Coates interviewed us on his syndicated TV show in November 1960. The show ran in six cities, and we received five hundred letters. By now OA had completely woven itself into the fabric of my life. I couldn't tell where marriage and motherhood ended and OA began. Excited by the telecast, I felt enormous hope for my recovery. Yet, I couldn't admit the uncertainty and fear that often overwhelmed me.

Right after the interview, Jim began urging me to reinstate AA's original Step Three. Stubbornly, I refused. "Listen Rozanne," he coaxed. "If you could have done it by yourself, you would have done it by yourself. But all your life you've depended on doctors, fad diets, and pills. These are all powers outside of you. Now," he went on, "you have a meeting every week, and you talk to someone every day. Don't you see that these are powers outside of you, too?" Reluctantly, I agreed.

His next few statements were to alter my life forever. "Rozanne," he persisted, "suppose you take the capital "p" off of Power and make it a small "p." Then say, 'I'm willpowerless over food.' Can you do that?" With that phrase, Jim had grabbed my attention. "Will power" was a dieter's term. All my life I'd said, "I have no will power." Now I could admit to being willpowerless over food without having to admit to a belief in a Higher Power. Without my realizing it, Jim had opened the door to a spiritual way of life for me. I couldn't step over that threshold yet, but the time was coming.

As a result of Jim's insistence, I gave in and wrote some new Twelve Steps. AA's Third Step was reinstated, but I still couldn't make all of our Steps identical to AA's Steps.

During the next two years my own inner conflicts increased. I was not overeating, I was thin, and I was a mass of self-will imposed on everyone. I felt that because I was slender and had been one of OA's founders that every word I uttered was a pearl of wisdom. Everyone ought to listen to me. That was the only way I could make myself feel important. I couldn't achieve that feeling from inside, and I simply didn't know what else to do.

Frequently I stepped on the toes of my fellow members, and they retaliated. Members began vilifying me in the meetings; some even telephoned to call me names. Late one Tuesday night a woman called to read me the riot act in no uncertain terms. Two nights later she did the same thing. She slammed her receiver down; I was helpless and horrified. I threw myself down on the floor in the darkened living room. Sobbing uncontrollably, I cried out, "God, if you're there, you've got me." And that's how I found the God of my understanding.

However, my recovery was only beginning. The resentment toward my mother, which I had carried for twenty-five years, was corroding my very core. "It's time for Steps Eight and Nine," said my sponsor, Thelma. At her prodding, I made amends to my parents. They lived in another city, so I had to write to them. I took the letter to the big mailbox on the corner and dropped it in. As I turned to walk away, I heard the heavy clank of the mailbox door. With that sound, twenty-five years of resentment disappeared. In one brief moment, everything was gone! I could hardly believe it; to me it was a miracle.

My next major step occurred early in 1962. In those days, and while I was growing up, calorie counting had been the dieter's mainstay. That's how I had learned to cut my food intake. It didn't matter how much I ate or how often, as long as my total food count remained within the limits I had set for myself. Unfortunately, nibbling on low-calorie vegetables between meals only increased my compulsion.

Although I'm not an alcoholic, during those early years I was attending AA meetings every week in order to learn more about the Twelve Steps and Twelve Traditions. Late in 1961, one powerful Sunday-noon AA meeting completely transformed my way of thinking about eating. Ordinarily, the AA's talked about sobriety. However, on this day the main speaker kept referring to "abstinence" from alcohol. This was the first time I'd ever heard sobriety referred to in that manner. It was a revelation!

Sitting in the back row, I said to myself, "That's what wrong with all of us in OA, including me. We're not abstaining from food during the day at all. Nibbling between meals is only reinforcing our obsession. Sometime during the day we have to 'abstain' from eating." Because I was a dietician's daughter, I recalled my mother's teachings about three meals a day.

At the next OA meeting, I was really excited. "Listen, everybody," I bubbled, "I have a new idea. With our between-meal nibbling, we're not abstaining from eating at all. That applies to me as well. We need to close our mouths from the end of one meal to the beginning of the next. I know we have to eat, so let's try three meals a day. We'll have nothing in between but no-calorie beverages, and we'll call that abstinence. If your doctor says more meals, the same principle will apply." Even then I knew abstaining referred not to the food plan itself but to the act of staying away from compulsive eating.

Some members thought it was an inspiration; others just laughed. But many members violently disagreed, and that's when the arguments began. I jumped right into the fight, and the negative excitement threatened to destroy my emerging serenity. However, I was still thin and going to meetings, so I believed I was safe from my disease.

In July 1964, after several inventories, I took one specifically on compulsive spending. On July 30, when I brought the inventory to my sponsor's house, I weighed 109 pounds. I walked out of Thelma's home believing that I would never spend like that again. I walked right into a family party, took that first bite and continued to overeat.

A year later, although my overspending had stopped, my eating was out of control, and I'd gained seventeen pounds with no end in sight. Terrified at what was happening to me, I resigned as national secretary. Luckily, Margaret P., a former executive secretary, stepped in to take my place.

Six years later Margaret died of cancer, and I came back to fill her job. Unfortunately, I was fat and getting fatter. By late April 1972, I was back to 148 pounds. The trustees fired me as OA's national secretary. They felt that everyone representing OA at the national level had to be a physical example of recovery. To save face, I submitted a letter of resignation, citing ill health and family pressures.

Years later I came to appreciate the value of the trustees' actions. They had not enabled my disease. They had insisted on recovery on all three levels for OA national service workers, and they were absolutely right. I will be forever grateful to them for this valuable lesson.

At that time, however, self-pity overwhelmed me. I took that firing as a personal rejection. Somehow, the essence of the OA program was eluding me, and only food could ease my misery. By the following year, my body ballooned to 185 pounds. Confusion and despair filled my life.

Yet, one blessing remained—I kept coming back to meetings. Sitting in the back of the room, I felt hopeless and desolate, unable to make a phone call when I wanted to eat. Compulsive overeating is a disease of isolation, and my paralyzing inability to call was part of my illness.

Finally, one hot summer night in 1973, I heard a speaker, Cynthia L., whom I'd never seen before. Approaching her after the meeting, I told her I was leaving OA, that this was my last meeting.

The next morning she called me. "Hi, Rozanne, I just wanted to tell you I love you." Cynthia called me every day for weeks. She loved me because I was a member of the human race, not because I was thin or had achieved anything marvelous. Her simple acceptance of me kept me in Overeaters Anonymous.

The next years were a great learning experience for me. Although I began to lose weight very slowly, incomprehensible demoralization was still a part of my daily life. I kept coming back to OA, and I certainly learned a lot about patience. Yet the ability to love myself still eluded me; my heart was clouded with self-hate.

One day in late 1978 during an OA convention meeting, I heard a speaker, Mary, tell her story. As she ended, she said, "I tried to tell myself, 'Mary, you're okay,' and I couldn't say it in front of a mirror. It took me six months to do it."

Later that night I bragged to myself, "I can certainly do that right now." But I couldn't. I tried to tell myself I was okay, and I started to cry. Then I remembered my sponsor's lessons. Thelma had taught me to "act as if." She told me that I didn't have to want it, or like it, or believe it. "Just take the action," she had urged, "and the feelings will follow."

Acting as if it were true, I practiced telling myself, "Rozanne, you're okay." Unable to look at myself in the mirror, I said this phrase all day, every day for six months. Then one December evening, I was dressed for a party. In a hurry to leave, I paused briefly to check myself in the hall mirror before rushing out the door. Then I suddenly stopped and looked at myself. I smiled and said, "Rozanne, you're okay. You are one fantastic lady, and I love you." That wondrous feeling has remained with me to this day, evidence of God's work in my life.

By late 1979 I weighed 137. My family doctor had given me an antidepressant to ease my ever-present headaches, but that particular drug had an unfortunate side effect. It caused weight gain. By September 1981, I was back to 172 pounds. Luckily, an eating-disorder specialist discovered my plight and took me off the drug. With that action, some of my overeating lessened and twenty-five of my excess pounds disappeared.

But still I struggled. Abstaining for short periods, I would give in and overeat again. What was wrong? I prayed for a miracle, terrified that I might be an OA failure, ashamed to return to meetings. Yet I knew there was nowhere else for me to go, and so I kept coming back. Little by little, I gained weight again.

By spring of 1986 I weighed 171 pounds. Then slowly I began to abstain from the worst of my compulsive overeating. There were still slips, but surrender gradually entered my heart. I began to truly realize that I was a compulsive overeater who couldn't control her eating alone. I wasn't bingeing as I had in the past; I wasn't eating between my planned meals. Again I prayed for help. Suddenly, the unexpected happened.

In January 1987, the Los Angeles Intergroup had its annual OA birthday party. A.G., my longtime friend from Texas, had returned to OA after an eighteen-year absence. He had been the first man in OA in 1962. He had lost over 100 pounds and had been chairman of our first Board of Trustees. Then, like so many, he had left OA and regained the weight.

By January 1987, this wonderful man had been back in OA for a year. He was maintaining his normal weight and working the Steps. He came to Los Angeles from his Texas home to join in the birthday celebration.

He and my husband, Marvin, and I went out to dinner each night, taking turns paying the bill. One fateful night A.G. took a piece of paper out of his pocket and began writing.

"What are you doing?" I protested. "It's our turn to pay the bill."

He shook his head and continued writing. "I'm counting my calories," he replied.

His comment stayed with me all through that night. My treasured friend had what I wanted. He had a slender body, and more important, his eyes had a light that could only come from spiritual recovery.

"If he can make it, I can make it," I told myself. "I grew up counting calories. That's not so scary; I can do that."

Praying for guidance, I asked God for an eating plan I could live with the rest of my life. "Through health and illness, through travel and at home, through parties, bar mitzvahs, holidays and ordinary days, help me to nourish my body with the right food in the proper amounts." Then I said, "However long it takes to lose this weight is however long it's going to take."

The next day I sat down to write an eating plan for myself. Allowing for several health problems, my age, height, and daily activities, I arrived at a nourishing plan for myself, with abstinence from food between my allotted meals.

That day I began to weigh and measure everything I ate. I hadn't been bingeing in my old manner, but I was appalled at how much I'd been consuming. No wonder I was still fat! At my short height, I was eating too much for my body.

By the third day of this new plan I began to feel a lightening of my spirit, as if an inner weight were being lifted. It was so beautiful, I knew at once it was hope. For the first time in years, I could see the light at the end of the tunnel. Because I'd been going to meetings for twenty-seven years, I understood that I would have to work those Twelve Steps immediately. No matter how effective my eating plan was, weighing and measuring alone just wouldn't work. My salvation lay in those Steps.

I had long ago learned that eating plans and meetings are not my program of recovery. Although they are helpful and even necessary, AA's "Big Book" statement was more than ever true for me: "Here are the Steps which are suggested as a program of recovery."

Since 1961 I've taken twenty-four Fourth Steps and hundreds of Tenth Steps. Today I continue to surrender, make amends, carry the OA message, and practice these principles in all my affairs.

Beginning in 1962, I've had a period of prayer and meditation every morning before I start my day. It's become a habit, one which has stood me in good stead as I surrendered myself to my Higher Power each day and admitted my powerlessness over food.

Since our recovery is spiritual, emotional, and physical, I'm careful to include a daily routine of exercise and walking. It took three years to lose forty pounds. That slow weight loss allowed my mind to become thin along with my body. (On other diets, I'd lost weight so fast that my head stayed fat while my figure slenderized.)

Because I pay attention to what goes into my mouth, I can pay attention to what goes into my heart and mind and soul. Today I can enjoy a normal-size body while maintaining a sixty-pound weight loss from my top weight.

Instead of being a struggle, life is really fun! I delight in spending time with my husband and with my daughters and their husbands. I can take pleasure in playing with my small grandsons and appreciate working in my beautiful rose garden.

I care about others because I care about myself. Because I kept coming back, I learned the validity of an elementary spiritual principle given to me by the Reverend Rollo M. Boas, one of OA's earliest supporters: If you remove your body from the truth, when you are ready, the truth is nowhere to be found. But if you continue to bring your body to the truth, then when you are ready, the truth is waiting there for you."

And that truth—our promise of recovery—is in every OA meeting when we join hands, pray together, and joyously, lovingly encourage one another: Keep coming back!

A loving tribute . . .

Since this story was written, a heart attack took my beloved husband, Marvin, on November 11, 1999. Many of you knew him well. Most of you have heard me praise his patience, support, and encouragement during OA's first forty years. He took care of our babies when Jo S. and I met during that first year. He strengthened and sustained me when I set up an office in our little dining room. He joined us—you and me—at birthday parties, conferences, and conventions, always sharing in our trials and triumphs. He believed in us and what we were trying to achieve. Marvin was our earliest and most faithful friend, and we will all miss his loving, gentle presence.

For more on the history of Overeaters Anonymous, read *Beyond Our Wildest Dreams*, available from the WSO.

2

He Never Let a Hot Doughnut Get Cold

MY CLASSMATES CALLED ME "Blubber" in grammar school, and I hated them for it. I cannot hear the word used even in its proper context today, almost sixty years later, without a stab of pain. My parents realized I had a problem when I was about seven, and I then began what was to become a lifetime of visits to doctors.

The pediatrician was a friend of my mother's; he said she shouldn't worry, that I'd probably outgrow my weight problem. Having heard many times that obesity is the result of sin, I wonder what sins I had committed at age four or six that had made me so fat. (Most of the juicy, fun sins hadn't even crossed my mind at that time.)

An early OA member and friend of mine used to say, "On every school playground, there is at least one fat child, and on my playground, it was me." I was the fat one on my playground, fatter than the merely plump ones, the butt of all the jokes and jibes. I used to wish that I had been born deformed or crippled, because at least others tried to help those unfortunates.

But they only laughed at me, implying that it was my fault I was fat. That hurt me so deeply because I believed it was true. Occasionally, I hear OA members say they are glad to be compulsive eaters, because that makes them eligible for this wonderful program. I can't believe they were fat children. I love what this program does for me, too, but I wouldn't go through the hell of being a fat child again for anything.

I attended several schools as a child, each one a new place for bullies to use me as a target. In high school, my nickname was "June Bug," after the huge, repulsive beetle with lots of tiny legs. I graduated about four months after my sixteenth birthday, at 287 pounds. As you can guess, I wasn't very popular with the girls. That sense of always being on the outside of things left scars that still trouble me.

I went away to college and began isolating for the first time. I started to eat compulsively in grand style there, gaining weight so rapidly that my skin couldn't keep up; I still have stretch marks from my elbows to my knees. (I never wear short sleeve shirts, even now. Yet, my stretch marks serve as a reminder of exactly how I would be today were it not for this miraculous program.)

While in college, I went to a bakery every morning at about three o'clock when the hot doughnuts were ready. I bought eighteen doughnuts, a Boston cream pie, and a half gallon of milk. I always ate the doughnuts on the way back to my room. A fitting epitaph for my tombstone would be, "Here Lies a Man Who Never Let a Hot Doughnut Get Cold!" For most people, college is one of the high points in life: new friends, independence, interesting courses. My eating and my inability to handle the vagaries of life made me a failure in college. I left after a couple of years, just in time to avoid expulsion.

Once during this period, my doctor checked my blood pressure and immediately put me in the hospital, where I remained for six weeks. My blood pressure was normal after a few hours of quiet and rest, but they realized I needed to lose weight more than anything else. They kept me there, and believe it or not their diet worked! I lost weight. Then they made a critical error—allowing me to leave. I regained the weight, plus a few extra pounds.

Soon I was married and began another round of medical exams. I discovered amphetamines, and I loved them. I could control my eating while high, work twenty-four hours a day, talk a blue streak, and feel wonderful until I collapsed about three days later. Then I'd gorge myself and sleep the whole thing off. I believe I've been on every diet known to humankind, and I saw each one as my marvelous solution, even when I repeatedly didn't lose weight.

All this led to my first visit with a psychiatrist. After a session or two, he told me that the easiest way for him to help me was for me to go lose the weight, then we could discuss whatever problems were unearthed. I thought it a great idea and left to do just that. I paused on the way home, though, to pick up a cheeseburger and a chocolate malt. He may as well have advised me to jump out the sixth-floor window and fly around the building before he would help me. He meant well.

I've spent countless hours eating while asking myself, "Why in the hell don't you quit?"

I knew I was full, but I needed just a little more to satisfy my elusive itch. The closest I came in my exhaustive search was a blend of sweet tastes with salty—as in peanut butter and jelly sandwiches with corn chips. (I tell my alcoholic friends they've never really known a bad morning aftertaste until they've had a peanut-butter hangover.)

From time to time, I vomited, but never on purpose. When I ate, I intended for it to stay down, but sometimes I ate so much my stomach couldn't contain it. I've spent entire nights on the bath mat so I wouldn't have to get out of bed to vomit again. And as soon as I had that relieved feeling, I thought I'd better eat a little something extra to keep from feeling weak. I was off again.

Asking a compulsive eater like me to diet is akin to offering someone ten dollars to not think of the word "hippopotamus" for the next five minutes. The harder I tried, the more impossible it became. I always thought everyone else wanted to eat the way I did, but they had the will power to control it. So my problem, as I saw it, was lack of will power. I did wonder why it was that I seemed to have enough will power to master several difficult things, yet still couldn't control the way I ate.

I'd been told, "Hell, even a dog knows when to quit eating." Well, it seems dogs have something I don't have; although, I have known one dog who didn't know how to quit. I had to hold him during feedings so he wouldn't choke. So not all dogs know. And neither did I.

Among the many things I tried was going to church. I don't mean to belittle religion, since it is how the majority of the world's people find and develop their spirituality, but it didn't work for me. I was told, "You'll get out of it what you put into it," so I went to work. I was there almost every time the door opened. I was on the governing board, headed the annual fund drive, and taught Sunday School, all to no avail. Someone said that I was praying for the wrong things. Perhaps I was. I kept asking God to take this monkey off my back, promising Him lots of things were He to do that. But as I saw it then, He didn't do His part.

However, church led me to a retreat on May 20, 1961, with two others in my car—one of them a recovering alcoholic with over two years of sobriety in the AA program. I finally got the courage to ask him if he thought AA might help me. I asked in a joking manner, so if he laughed I could laugh along with him. He paused a long time, and said, "I don't see why not."

He had heard the pain in my voice and, through him, God responded. He began to tell me a little about the program, and I instantly understood that this man wanted to drink for the same reasons I wanted to eat and that he had been able to refrain from drinking, happily, for over two years. Whatever had done that for him was exactly what I needed and wanted.

We stopped at my favorite German bakery on the way home, and I bought my usual bag of goodies. We talked all the way home, and that night my friend gave me my first chip, with the simple instruction that I was to throw it away where I couldn't ever find it again before breaking my diet. To this day I still carry a chip in my pocket.

During the twenty-four hours that followed, I underwent an overwhelming spiritual experience that has changed my life every day since, abstinent or not. The Steps didn't do it; I didn't know much about them at that point. What did it for me was that someone had been willing to give to me what had worked for him. Remember the bag of goodies from the German bakery? I never took the first bite.

John, my alcoholic sponsor, did tell me about "one day at

a time," and suggested that I make a daily contract with God, as I understood Him. I did so (and still do), asking God to relieve me of the compulsion to eat for this day and all the days of my life. The twenty minutes I spent in this way each morning, alone and quiet, made every day better. John began to take me through the Steps, explaining that they are "suggested," just as it's suggested that I not hold my head under water for five minutes.

After thirty-four days of continuous abstinence, I made my first Twelfth-Step call on my neighbor, Norma B. I was sure she was like I was. Norma was interested, began the program, and lost lots of weight. Together we formed Gluttons Anonymous. Our basic strength, however, came from AA, although neither of us was alcoholic. We were welcomed at both open and closed meetings and retreats, for which I will be forever grateful to them. They kept us on course while we tried to attract members to Gluttons Anonymous. In a little over a year, there were five Gluttons Anonymous groups in the Central Texas area.

In June 1962, we heard about Overeaters Anonymous through the AA office in New York. One Sunday night, at our regular Gluttons Anonymous meeting, I called Rozanne. She was gracious and made it clear that they were doing just as we were, using the Twelve Steps to recover from compulsive eating. Having felt so alone, we were delighted to find others following the program we were using. Further conversations led to a discussion about the upcoming first Conference, and representatives from each of our groups attended. Five delegates attended from GA and sixteen from OA. Therefore, the vote on the name of the newly merged organization was sixteen to five in favor of Overeaters Anonymous.

I became very active, devoting much of my time to OA matters. I knew the Steps by heart and was convinced that no one was more spiritual than I. On that basis, I made nearly four years of abstinence. Then the compulsion returned, and I slipped. I resigned my posts in OA and began to try to get back on the program. I was sure it would be easy, since I was so spiritual. Not so. Then I decided that the reason God had abandoned me was that my life wasn't "clean" enough. So I set out to clean it up, so He would again bless me. It didn't work. In fact, I was even more miserable due to my failure at perfection.

My weight was soaring. Once during that period, I put together eighty-five days of abstinence. But, to use the AA term, I was dry rather than sober. My weight went up and down. Then came the final surge, in which I gained over 100 pounds. I continued to go to meetings for four years; in March 1968, I decided that it was never going to work for me and I should just give it up. I boxed all my OA materials, sealed the box, and put it away.

As an old friend in the program used to say, "I carried an extra hundred pounds all day and even slept with it at night." I don't know what my top weight was, because I never had a scale that weighed over 300 pounds, but I know it exceeded that. I again tried all the fad diets and the new diet pills. I returned to psychotherapy, which was to last twenty years. The latter did help me in some respects, but did nothing for my weight.

I repeatedly asked my psychiatrist, "How long do you think it will be before I can start losing weight?" He would look at my chart, think for a moment, then respond, "I think in about six months." In twenty years there are forty six-month periods. It never happened.

Several things stayed with me from the program. The best part was that I never lost my understanding of a Higher Power. I knew He was there, but out of my reach. The worst thing was that I had enjoyed almost four years as a normal-sized person; it was especially difficult, at this point, to return to being a fat man.

In the fall of 1985, I answered the telephone at home one evening, and a man introduced himself as a member of OA. I was polite, but not cordial. He went on to tell me he had just returned from California where he'd attended an OA meeting, and that Rozanne had asked him to try to find me in Texas. (He was from Dallas.) She told him that she was writing the OA history and needed some information from me.

I agreed that I would call her, and a day or two later did so. Rozanne and I had always been friends, and the conversation was pleasant. I offered to send her some of my old files, wished her well, hung up the phone, and tried to forget the whole thing. I was on a new binge, unable to find anything that would satisfy my hunger, even for a moment.

I heard a radio talk show mention a new center in the beautiful hill country near San Antonio that held silent retreats. I hungered for the silence I had tasted in the AA retreats I'd attended. A few days later, I was in touch with the retreat center and found them willing to host a silent retreat for any size group, no matter how small. I decided that if I could get my former sponsor, now a drinking alcoholic, and the Episcopal priest who had encouraged my spiritual awakening during my abstinent days to go with me, I'd go. Of course, I hadn't seen or heard from either of them in years, so I was quite confident they wouldn't or couldn't go.

Wrong again. They were both delighted with the idea. I used the twenty-four hours of silence to read the "Big Book" and to decide if I should try the OA program once more. The decision seemed easy, and I immediately began my new abstinence. And, miracle of miracles, I made it through the first day without white-knuckling it!

When I returned home, I went to an OA meeting as soon as I could. I didn't use my real name for fear that someone from the early days might remember me; I didn't want another failure chalked up to my account. I was at a meeting when I had eight days of abstinence, and when it came my turn to speak, I said my name, that I was a glutton and compulsive eater, and that I had just witnessed eight personal miracles in a row. Now, more than ten years later, I still think of one day of abstinence as one miracle.

As of today, I have lost over 100 pounds and have maintained that loss for well over ten years. I lack the words to express my gratitude for this recovery. Life hasn't been completely smooth during this time, either. Since returning to OA, the following events have taken place in my life: significant weight loss; separation from my wife of thirty-seven years; sale of my business and a move from my home of thirty years; divorce, which divided the world into two camps—those who thought I was a bastard, and me; and my mother died. These events will be at the top of any list of stress values, but I didn't have to eat over any of them. This is not to say there was no pain; sometimes the pain was overwhelming, but I did not have the compulsion to eat.

Often I'm asked if I can look back and see why I slipped. Yes, I can. It was because I failed to use the last phrase of the Twelfth Step—to practice these principles in all my affairs. It was relatively easy to work the program on gluttony because I hated every aspect of it, and it ceased being fun so long ago, I can't even remember it. But as for lust and grandiosity, the problems were more difficult to identify because there was still some pleasure left in them for me. The program didn't work for me because I didn't work all of it: every phrase of every Step in every aspect of my life.

I've come to identify "bottom" as that point when one realizes that no combination or quantity of food will scratch the compulsive itch. I spent a lot of time looking, and I never did find it.

I've learned a new way to identify all my compulsive urges. For example, hunger is easily satiable, while a compulsion to eat is insatiable. With lust and grandiosity, the same principles apply for me. I try to use the "satiability test" on all my activities. I'm quite far from perfection in this area, but I've progressed light years from my starting point.

I'm having some new sensations in this second tour through the program. Many times, I've heard people say, "That's such a rich sauce, I can't eat but a bite of it." I always thought that was the most ridiculous thing I'd ever heard, since there was no such thing as a food that would slow me down. Now that's different. If I encounter a particularly rich food, a bite or two kills my appetite. Often I don't eat my full daily allotment of food merely because I am full and don't want it.

Is it possible that I was born with the same control mechanisms everyone else has, and that I overrode them for so long that atrophy took over? Could it be that after several years of abstinence they are becoming effective again? I don't understand the process, but I do feel it happening, and it's wonderful.

Yes, I still have days when all is not bright and cheery. I get angry with God, usually because He seems to refuse to let me see the big picture so I can understand everything. On a recent day when I was upset with Him for that reason, I entered the lane to my house from the road and opened my gate from the car with an automatic opener. As the gate swung open in front of me, a group of ten or fifteen young cows stood watching nearby. They didn't notice that I didn't have to get out and open the gate. Even had they been aware, I couldn't ever explain to them how it worked, coded transmitter and all.

The thought struck me that maybe this is the way it is between me and God. Perhaps it's all around me, and there is no need to explain it. The limitations of time and space make it impossible for me to see and understand God's magnitude.

I express my overwhelming gratitude for this program in many ways; one of them is writing this story so you can determine if you are as I was. If you think you are, welcome. This marvelous program will work for you, just as it has for me.

3

She Found
Herself

I HEARD ABOUT OA in 1961. I'd just had a nervous breakdown. I had lost some weight during the time I was depressed, but started to put it back on when my appetite returned and I was eating everything that wasn't bolted to the floor.

The year before, I had been in bed for three months threatening to abort my second child. Then my father died, my grandmother died, and I gave birth. During that year, I had never shed a tear. My psychiatrist said I had a war raging inside me until the dam finally broke. I started to cry and couldn't stop. I cried day and night for four weeks. I was in such bad shape my husband had to hire a nurse to take care of my two daughters—one an infant and one a two-year-old. I couldn't even hold a baby bottle. But I always told you I was fine! I could solve your problems and give you good advice, but I could never apply it to myself.

I didn't come to OA immediately after I heard about it. The only meeting in Los Angeles was in the evening, and I was afraid to drive at night, so I stayed home. One night the secretary of the group called and asked if I would pick up another member who didn't have a car and bring her to the meeting. So another compulsive overeater brought me to my first meeting.

What I heard at that meeting changed my life. They shared about secret binges, eating in the car, using food to push down feelings. I had done the same things. For the first time in my life, I didn't feel like a freak. I wasn't alone anymore.

Six months after joining OA, in September 1961, we moved to the San Fernando Valley. There were two meetings in the valley at that time. I played around with the program for a long time. After two and a half years, though I had lost some weight, I was doing in OA what I had done outside of OA: abstaining from Monday to Friday and bingeing on the weekends. I was tired of it. That is when I met my first sponsor.

She was a recovering alcoholic, and she believed she had also found the answer to the obsession with food. She wanted me to follow a specific plan—no sugar or carbohydrates while I worked the Twelve Steps. I said I would.

A group of us went to an old hotel in downtown LA to listen to a man discuss working the Twelve Steps. I listened intently. I was determined for the first time in my life to accomplish something. Most of my life I had been a great starter but never seemed to finish anything. All those half-finished afghans and sweaters attested to that. I wanted to do as little work as possible in life and get great results. That philosophy hadn't worked up to this time. Then I remembered the passage from Chapter 5 of the "Big Book": "Rarely have we seen a person fail who has thoroughly followed our path." I had never done anything thoroughly in my life, but in April 1964 I decided to do exactly that—to give my all to saving my own life.

I launched into reading and learning about the Steps. I took Step Two, even though I didn't think I was insane, but my sponsor reminded me that the definition of insanity was "doing the same thing over and over and expecting different results." I had certainly done that with dieting and with other failures in my life. So I took Step Two on faith, followed by Step Three. I had no concept of a Higher Power, but used my sponsor and the group in that capacity.

My sponsor reminded me that a decision is not a decision unless it is immediately followed by action. She told me about the three birds sitting on a wire. Two of them decided to fly away. How many birds were left on the wire?" she asked. "Three," she answered, "because they only decided to fly away." So I wrote my Fourth Step hesitantly. It took me three months and filled a large spiral notebook.

When it came time to give it away, I chose someone I would never see again—an alcoholic recovering in AA. He wasn't surprised or judgmental, but told me he was only the "ears of God." When he asked me if I was entirely ready to have all my defects of character removed, I said, "Yes. Take them all." I'd completed Step Six. We both knelt and recited the Seventh-Step Prayer from page 76 of the "Big Book," and to my surprise two of my biggest defects were immediately removed: my obsession with food and my shoplifting.

I stole almost every day of my life. I usually took little things, but sometimes big items, as well. Every day I woke up and said, "Today I am going on a diet, and I'm not going to steal." Before dark, I had broken one or both of those oaths. What a relief, what a miracle to be free of these defects! I haven't eaten compulsively or stolen since April 1964.

Steps Eight and Nine were very scary for me, as I had a lot of amends to make. My sponsor reminded me that I was willing to go to any lengths to recover. I was scared, but willing. I chose a department store as my first of many amends. I didn't know anyone who had made such an amends, but I was determined to get well. I called the store, made an appointment with the manager, kissed my husband goodbye, and told him he might get a phone call to post bail. I didn't know if they locked people up for admitting shoplifting and returning to the scene of the crime. I told the store manager I was in a Twelve-Step program and this was part of my recovery. I had my check in my hand, but he didn't want to accept it.

I was the first person who had ever returned money to them. They had received anonymous checks in the mail and merchandise left at the doors before the store opened, but never a real, live person with a check in hand. I insisted they take the check. They congratulated me and introduced me around the corporate offices as though I were a celebrity. When I left, I felt ten feet tall. For the first time in my life, I liked who I was. I then went on to complete all my personal and financial amends.

I now believe that the Fourth through the Ninth Steps are there to remove all the things that prevent me from experiencing the "sunlight of the spirit." When those obstacles are removed, I see that I wasn't a bad person, just a misguided one.

I practice Steps Ten, Eleven, and Twelve daily. I now take

a Tenth Step each night before I go to sleep and do Step Eleven in the morning. I say the Third- and Seventh-Step Prayers each morning also. I need to get me out of the way and allow my Higher Power to direct my day.

Step Twelve empowers me to give to the world daily only a small part of what I have received from this program. When I recently wrote another Fourth Step, there were two questions at the end of the inventory. "If you died today, what do you think would be on your tombstone?" and "What would you like your tombstone to say?" I thought a long time and wrote in answer to number one, "Loving wife, mother, and daughter." And to number two, "She made a difference in other people's lives."

This program has given me the joy, hope, understanding, and help one compulsive eater can give to another. Before this program, I not only didn't know who I was and what my purpose in life could be, I didn't want to be me. I wanted to be someone else. I didn't like my looks, my body, my intellect, or any part of me. I wanted what you had—your hair, eyes, and personality. Today, I can truly say I like me. I have found myself. I was once lost to myself and my own life.

I am grateful to be a compulsive overeater, because without that symptom I would never have chosen this path to find out who I was. I used food to hide from me. I was afraid of what I would find if I looked. What I found surprised me. I found a truly wondrous person, one I am proud of!

4

Abstinence, Not Perfection

"I KNOW. I REALLY do know what it's like. And there is a solution." Those are the words that ushered me out of a denial driven by hopelessness into the path of my recovery. His name was Bill. He was a man, like me. He was middle-aged, like me. He was highly educated, like me. And he starved himself, like me. When he said that he had found a way out of his problem, I had hope that there might be a way out of the hell in which I was trapped.

At that point in my life, food and thoughts of food owned me. Controlling food was the most important thing I did. Nothing, absolutely nothing, was going to get in the way of my total control of food. My wife wasn't. My children weren't. My job wasn't. Nothing. I had quit going to restaurants and had started refusing to even come to the table if certain "disgusting" foods were served. As a couple, we had no social life (you never know when foods might show up), and as a family we had no picnics, no dinners out, no family gatherings. Avoiding all contact with food was my absolute rule. Taking my running clothes along to the church picnic was the closest I could come to social time with my family. Then, after a minimum appearance, I could change for a run home as my daily exercise. I was terrified that even being around food would cause me to become obese.

Did I think I had a problem? Yes, I thought I was probably a compulsive overeater who couldn't control his eating. At my lowest weight, people suggested that I might be anorexic. I laughed in their faces. I thought I was fat. I thought I was disgusting. I wasn't female; I wasn't a teenager. I thought anorexics were thin because they forgot to eat; I thought about food every waking moment of my life. I wished I were "anorexic."

At the time, I knew I had been "fat" all my life. My mother was "fat," and, by association, I had to be too. I had learned that food was dirty, and the less you handled it or ate it, the purer you were. While I knew and believed these things, I never acted on them until my thirty-first year. In that year, my younger sister committed suicide. I believed that my imperfections and flaws had kept me from being able to save her. I got up on New Year's Day 1980 and resolved to lose weight and exercise until I liked what I saw in the mirror. I nearly died, but I never once liked whom I saw. "Lose ten more pounds, and then you'll look okay," I would tell myself.

Then one day my wife called me at work to say she was leaving me. "I can't stop you from starving yourself, and I can't bear the thought of waking up one morning and finding you cold and dead next to me." I was stunned. I was getting thinner, better, purer. She was supposed to like me more this way. I promised to stop starving, and that persuaded her to stay.

Did this moment of crisis lead me to OA and recovery? No. I concluded that she had a problem, but that keeping her was important enough that I would force myself to eat more if that was what it took. My weight went up slightly, and I hated myself and resented her even more.

Four long years passed in that limbo state. Not able to use food the way I desperately wanted, I used alcohol more and more to numb the self-loathing. My loss of control with alcohol propelled me into a treatment center, yet my wife was afraid that I would sober up and return to starving. As for my attitude, I left for the center with my running clothes packed and every intention of teaching my body a lesson in purity through exercise and starvation.

There I met Bill; I was not alone. Through him, I experienced the unconditional love that is part of carrying the message to those who still suffer. I can't emphasize this enough. Information did not bring me to OA; identification did. I knew the Twelve Steps; my wife had been in OA for years. I had all the information necessary for a lifetime of recovery. But it was Bill's caring that gave me my belief in the Steps as a solution for me.

I was encouraged to make OA a part of my life and to do the things that are suggested, so I started with a clear, intuitive sense of what abstinence was for me. I was told to embrace the Third Tradition in claiming my membership in OA if anyone ever questioned me. Bill was 400 miles away, and within several months I lost all the simple clarity I had started with. My abstinence wasn't good enough or pure enough to impress anybody in OA, and I was so afraid of rejection that I dared not be honest about my anorexia in meetings. Six months after starting, I was lost, confused, and back into controlled eating.

I was controlling to a more moderate level, but the old obsession was back.

I found myself back with Bill during a Family Week program, and I shared my sense of loss and confusion with him. "What went wrong? The harder I worked my abstinence, the more obsessed I got." His answer? "Maybe the abstinence you want isn't the right abstinence for you. Knowing you, here is what I might suggest . . ." Let there be no doubt that I did not want the abstinence he suggested; there was no purity or painful self-sacrifice in it. Well, I tried it, as much to show him that it wouldn't work as anything. That was over ten years ago, and it has worked just fine.

I've learned many things from this experience with abstinence. First, as a newcomer to OA I was seeking guidance from a very sick person—me—concerning my abstinence. A sponsor with whom I had shared a Fifth Step had much clearer insight into my disease than I did. Second, I can always trust the power of the disease. While my abstinence is unique to me, I was not free to choose whatever I wanted it to be. If I choose an abstinence that lets me "feed the dragon," the "dragon" will get stronger. So today when I wonder, "Is my abstinence right?" I can remind myself that I'm not powerful enough to fool my compulsion. I have been essentially free of the food obsession, free of having to control my eating, and have been at the same healthy weight for over ten years. It works. I will be forever grateful that Bill encouraged me, and that I had just enough willingness to try it.

This abstinence has not changed since the start, because my disease has not been cured. My abstinence is firmly anchored to my First Step and in refusing participation in the self-abuse that almost killed me. From time to time, I have been tempted to expand my abstinence to include things that have to do with attaining complete balance and perfection in my eating habits, my relationships, and my job. Yes, I want that balance in my life, but my old black-and-white thinking pushes me to the conclusion that changing my plan of eating is the way I make all the changes in my life. Now I have many tools, and so today I ask for God's help in each of the things I want for my life. But I leave my abstinence alone.

Bill also encouraged me to get and stay totally honest about my anorexia in meetings. "Find out what they will really do," he said. "You've already judged them in your mind by withholding your honesty. Why not give them a chance to speak for themselves?" I went back and identified myself as anorexic up front, and nothing happened. I think somehow they already knew. My OA brothers and sisters and I have discovered a richness of identification in recovery that has benefited us all.

Several years ago, for example, two of my friends and I did an exciting panel at a region convention called, "Same Disease, Different Symptoms." It was a powerful experience of the unity we had come to feel as compulsive eaters. I've sustained this connectedness over the years through service. "Don't just attend the meetings, join OA," Bill had said. I did. Being "a part of" happened because I made the coffee, and then I became group secretary, then was treasurer, then worked on the convention, and on and on. I belong in OA, and I now know that fact deeply in my heart because of the love and acceptance I have experienced here.

Things are now immensely better with my family, my friends, and my coworkers. My relationships didn't seem to improve much during the first several years, though. It was only after getting abstinent that I began to see how badly I'd behaved. I was overwhelmed, but I did what my sponsor suggested: I worked the Steps. He told me that the word "amends" in the Eighth and Ninth Steps was the same word as an "amendment" to the Constitution. It meant a change, not just an apology. So I changed the way I treated my wife, my children, and all those in my life. I approached them for my Ninth Step to tell them that they deserved better than I had given, and that the old ways were no longer acceptable to me. Things steadily changed.

Two years into abstinence, I looked at my wife and said, "I don't know if we're going to make it." She answered, "I don't know, either." How ironic that now my recovery was more important than staying married, when years before I had promised to change my eating just to keep her from leaving. In putting our own recoveries first, we gave each other the space to build a healthy relationship. We've been on that bumpy road for several years now. To me, this is proof that my God is doing for me what I could not do for myself.

With my children, I have been available to parent my way through some very difficult times. I was told early on that there were no points for style, and as a parent, I exemplify that. My children are grown now, but what I cherish about my abstinent years of parenting is that today those two grown daughters are both on a spiritual path, at least partly because they have seen what a difference God can make in another person's life. A key word in all these relationships for me is dignity. These people get the real and honest me to live with and work with, someone who is willing to listen, to share, and to change when needed.

I think of myself as a newcomer to OA whose life is just

beginning to take off. I've felt that way from the start. Each year takes me to places I never knew existed, and I glimpse possibilities I never imagined. Three words now define who I am and all that I do: honesty, dignity, and service. These are words whose meaning I have learned in Overeaters Anonymous. Thank you.

By the way: I know. I really do know what it's like. And there is a solution.

5 _____

The Miracle of the Twentieth Century

I WAS A CHILD of the great depression. I was in the third grade, a little over seven years old. When we were weighed by the school nurse, she bellowed out, "one hundred twenty-six pounds." Some children gasped and others snickered, but I do not remember ever feeling "fat" in my young years—just different.

I didn't see my mother as an obese woman either, but I do remember an episode when she took me shopping with her to buy a dress for herself. When the saleswoman asked her what size she was, Mom replied, "size fifty-two." I saw nothing wrong; I was just happy my mom was getting a new dress.

Looking back, I can see that I was happy on the outside, but crying on the inside. Things were difficult financially, and I began to take on many of my parents' fears. My overeating intensified during this period. When I was eight, we lost our home and moved to a small farm on the outskirts of town. It was rustic, to say the least. The house had no running water and had an outdoor toilet, but we tried to make the best of it. My dad was too proud to ask for public assistance, so seven of us lived there for two years, and then we moved back to town. Things improved a little, but my compulsive eating was in full swing. By the time I was seventeen, I weighed 230 pounds.

I went to nursing school at a most prestigious Boston hospital and excelled academically, but my weight changed very little during my student days. I was often lonesome; I had few friends and certainly no boyfriends. After I graduated, I began to go on diets—always losing weight and gaining it back again. I continued to do this for many years, occasionally attaining a normal weight.

In 1955, I married after a two-year courtship. I was twenty-eight years old and at a fairly normal weight. We had three children and then bought a home in the suburbs. My weight fluctuated up and down in what I have since learned to call the yo-yo syndrome, always ending up a little heavier than before. This continued in various forms until I came to Overeaters Anonymous at age forty, weighing over two hundred pounds and absolutely hating myself. I'd stopped smoking in May of that year and gained thirty pounds in ten weeks. I complained to a friend of mine that I wanted to lose weight. She said, "I don't understand how you gain all this weight. I never see you eat." What I didn't tell her was that I was a closet eater and looked forward to my binges when my husband and children went to bed. This same friend said she had recently seen an ad in the local paper about Overeaters Anonymous, and it gave a telephone number. No one in the East had ever heard of OA. I called the number the next day and spoke to a woman named Bernice; that was the beginning of a series of miracles that changed my life.

I'd promised myself many times that tomorrow I wouldn't do it again, a promise that lasted only until I went into the kitchen. Bernice understood perfectly what I was talking about, and we agreed to meet at her home. She had been trying to start an OA group after she had moved east from California, where OA was born in 1960.

Just the two of us were at that first meeting. (Today, I can say that God was there, as well!) We sat at her kitchen table, and she showed me how they did it in California. She read "How It Works." I felt strange because I heard God mentioned a few times. I thought to myself, "What did I get into here? This must be a cult of some sort. They always start in California and roll east!" Bernice intuitively understood my hesitation when I was leaving that first meeting. She introduced me to the infamous "gray sheet" diet and asked me to come back the next week. That's how it started for me. I never stopped coming back.

I began to listen and understand what abstinence was all about. These were all new concepts to me. What I was doing obviously wasn't working, as I was well over two hundred pounds at this time. I did try it, and I began to lose weight and feel better. After a few weeks, Bernice kept saying, "If we don't give it away, we won't be able to keep it ourselves." I didn't understand this concept either, but I went to see the minister of a local church and asked for the use of a meeting room. I put a notice in the local newspaper about an Overeaters Anonymous meeting.

No one had ever heard of it, but over fifty newcomers came to the first meeting. Bernice and I cried with joy, even though we had no literature. All we had to distribute were copies of the gray sheet that she had brought with her from California. The meeting grew very slowly at first, but people began to recover from compulsive overeating, including me. I was often disappointed when many of those who came in the early days never came back. Somehow or other, God kept me ·coming back week after week, even if occasionally I was the only one there.

I began to learn about what was really wrong with me. It was not only my obese body, but an emotional and a spiritual disease as well. I suffered from low-level, chronic depression at that time. I always felt better when I was on a diet, but I never was able to connect my eating to my moods. Neither was the psychiatrist I saw twice a week for several years. My therapist often said, "Tell me how you feel, and perhaps we can understand why you eat." How could I tell him how I felt when, on the way to therapy, I always stopped for a large ice cream cone and numbed out my feelings? In OA, I learned that we do just the opposite. We say, "Put the food down—no matter why you are eating. Get abstinent, and through a study of the Twelve Steps, you will come to understand why you ate compulsively."

I used to blame my mother for my obesity. It was her fault because when I went home to visit she made all of my favorite foods, and I never had the will power to resist. I always ate the food and yelled at her for making it. One of the first great gifts I received was the understanding that the eating was my responsibility. After a Fourth-Step inventory, followed by a series of amends, I was able to go to my mother and ask her to forgive me for my yelling at her and blaming her. I was able to tell her that she was really a wonderful mother and that I loved her very much. I was blessed that I was able to do this while she was alive; she died two years after I came into OA. She was a most loving mother, but my compulsive overeating interfered with our relationship. I was fortunate to have made those amends.

I began to change slowly in many other ways. My husband had told me that I was hard to live with. It was difficult for me to see that truth while my food was out of control, but after a period of abstinence, I was able to look at myself more honestly. If I disagreed with something, I could speak in a pleasant tone of voice and let him know that I did not share his point of view. If he spoke harshly to me, I could say, "It would mean a lot to me if you did not speak to me in that way." I had to look at what I was doing that irritated other members of my family and try to correct it. I asked for their forgiveness.

I recently found a letter that my then-eight-year-old son wrote to me describing perfectly what was going on in our home before I discovered this Fellowship. He wrote: "Dear Mommy, I thought that you said you would try not to yell at me and Anne and Ellen, but you still do yell. And I don't think you're trying not to yell. From, Mark." I cried when I came upon this letter recently. I took it to his home, showed it to him and his wife, and asked his forgiveness. I did not know when he was young how powerless and controlling I was with all my yelling, eating, and crying.

Incidentally, five months into the OA program, I saw the psychiatrist for the last time on a regular basis. When I told him I wanted to terminate, he said, "I never remember you looking this well. I don't know what you are getting from that group you attend, but it's something I am unable to give you."

I don't want anyone to think that I have had perfect abstinence for the past twenty-five years. I am not perfect. Today,

I do not have to be perfect. I describe my abstinence as "perfectly imperfect." I have made plenty of mistakes, but our recovery program has a well-documented list of things to do to take corrective action. These Twelve Steps are called "a design for living"; they work for the food problem and for any other type of problem. They are a great source of strength for me. They are the core of my recovery. This is definitely not a diet club!

I attend as many meetings as I can. I use all the tools. I may not have adhered perfectly to my plan of eating, but I consider my recovery perfect. God accepts me and loves me just the way I am. He is teaching me to do the same through the Twelve Steps. I am better able to accept and love other people just the way they are, without trying to change them and especially without being angry with them. This is such a gift of freedom. I lost about one hundred pounds, and the greatest miracle is that it has never been necessary for me to put that weight back on.

I have developed a wonderful relationship with a Higher Power. This is crucial; I cannot do it by myself. Every morning I ask my Higher Power to keep me abstinent, show me His will for today, and give me the power to carry it out—whatever it is. It is not always easy, especially when His will does not coincide with mine. I try to adopt a spiritual attitude and ask myself what God would like me to learn from my experiences. Is it a lesson in patience, or perhaps tolerance, or learning how to forgive someone who may have offended me? The end result of these spiritual exercises is that I have developed a new love and respect for myself. This allows me the greatest gift—to be able to accept and love others, exactly as they are.

I have learned to cope with difficult and painful situations with dignity and aplomb, through sharing my deepest feelings with other members of the Fellowship. A few years ago, for example, my brother and my husband died just a few days apart. I was able to share my pain with OA members who cared and listened with patience. They reminded me that food wouldn't bring my loved ones back to me. I kept sharing as my wounds healed. It was truly a miracle.

This program is the miracle of the twentieth century, in my mind. God knew from the beginning that I needed it. He led me here, even when I didn't know where I was going. All I can say is that my life really did begin at forty.

6

It's Elementary

When I began compiling photographs to demonstrate my history of obesity, my mother supplied pictures of me as a child. As she handed me one of my sister and me, she repeated the all-too-familiar phrase we had used in response when someone greeted us with "Hi, Fatty! Hi, Skinny!" My sister said, "I'm not skinny. I'm just slender, tender, and tall," while I said, "I'm not fat. I'm just pleasingly plump." I was surprised to notice a cute, round face looking back at me from the photograph. I wasn't fat at all; I was barely plump. Pictures from my teens also confirmed this.

I'd always felt fat, though, and was always dieting and stealing money to buy treats from the corner bakery. When I became old enough to baby-sit, my eating began in earnest. I got out of my abusive home and into a place where I could eat all I wanted. I still remember the humiliation of a neighbor telling my mother, "Your daughter is a wonderful baby-sitter, but boy, can she eat!" The effects of this compulsive eating didn't show up until I turned sixteen. By then, I had access to a car, more food, and freedom from my family.

Through my high school years, I binged and starved—starved all week and binged every weekend—and kept my weight in a normal range. But I always felt fat, and the "normal" range went higher and higher. After my first year at college, I weighed 190 pounds, so my mother took me to get diet pills at my Christmas break.

I continued to binge and starve, but got my weight down to 160 pounds for my wedding day. I was twenty years old and had just found someone to take care of me. I thought I was the luckiest girl alive.

After twenty years of superwife and supermom to six kids, I weighed 227 pounds. I'd tried liquid protein, shots, diet pills, and figure-control salons. They all worked wonders: I was fat one year and thin the next. As the years passed, I determined that I was good at bingeing and good at starving, but I was better at bingeing. I resigned myself to quit the diets and just be fat and happy. I had managed the fat. I just couldn't get the happy.

In OA I found people who understood how I ate. I hoarded food. I didn't like to share food. I planned events around food. I wanted some of everything, sometimes a lot of everything. I couldn't imagine how someone could eat three meals a day, day after day, and not be very obese. But I became willing to try.

My first plan of eating was three binges a day. I binged for fifteen minutes at breakfast, fifteen minutes at lunch and fifteen minutes at dinner. I didn't worry about what I ate, just when and for how long. And I was amazed. I lost weight bingeing! I became honest about how I really ate and started to see a correlation between how I felt and wanting to overeat.

One morning at around ten o'clock, I wanted to eat a candy bar. But I had made a commitment to abstinence, so I saved it to eat with my lunch. I can't say whether I actually ate it at lunch, but the important thing was that I stuck to my commitment not to eat in between meals. I eventually became willing to choose a healthy plan of eating that would allow me to lose weight, and I've adopted an exercise plan. For six years my weight has continued to go down.

How did that happen? It happened because, as I've heard so often in meetings, "Abstinence is the most important thing in my life today without exception." Without abstinence, I have nothing. That's why I go to Overeaters Anonymous. Because I don't want food to rule my life anymore, I must begin with abstinence—"an honest desire to stop eating compulsively." I was told that when I put down the food, I would have clarity, and I was astonished to find out it's true. Without the food, I was able to pause and think instead of reacting to situations.

I had been somewhat abusive, both physically and verbally, to my children. One time my husband said, "Didn't your father do that to you?" And I replied, "Yes." In his kind voice he said, without judgment, "Did you like it?" When I admitted I didn't, in fact, I hated him for it, he said, "Well, why would you do that to someone else?" It didn't make sense, but with the food, I just reacted. Without the food, I could choose how to act. As I looked up the word "serenity" in the dictionary—"clear, unclouded"—I knew what it meant because I'd been willing to give up the food.

I had been raised in a very religious home, but I questioned whether the God I supposedly loved was really there. My constant prayer (well, at least my Monday morning prayer) was, "Help me stay on this diet." Today I realize that such a prayer was a lie. I didn't want to stay on the diet; I just wanted to eat what I wanted to eat and be thin. I began to believe that a power greater than myself could restore me to sanity. When I finally made the decision to turn my will and my life over to the care of God as I understood Him, I thought big stuff was bound to happen. Every morning I prayed, "God, please remove my obsession with food today." And I added, "And let me know what you want me to do for you." I honestly listened to find out what it was He wanted me to do; I was sure it was going to be something magnificent.

The first thing I remember being impressed to do was to fasten my seat belt while driving. I always had a thousand rea- sons not to do so—"I'm almost home," "I haven't been in an accident yet," "It'll wrinkle my dress." But because I remem- bered I'd made a decision to turn my life and my will over to the care of God as I understood Him, I fastened the seat belt. I was awed by my instant sense of peace and well-being.

I began to practice listening more intently for ways I could be of service to God and my fellows. I finally "got it" one day when I had a strong urge to call my sister—the "slen- der, tender, and tall" one who now weighed over 300 pounds. My prayer had been, "Give me the courage and the willing- ness to do it," but I wasn't perfect, and I didn't want to call my sister. All day long I procrastinated, but the feeling persist- ed, and a few hours later I tried again. When she answered, she responded, "Oh, thank you so much for calling. I knew you wouldn't forget that my husband died a year ago today." I don't always have to figure out how to serve God. He will let me know what to do.

Step Four was a challenge, but by now I was convinced the program was working. I was losing weight, I was feeling worthwhile, and I was beginning to be happy. So I did it, and I gave it away (Step Five). I identified my character defects (Step Six), and I asked God to remove them all (Step Seven) before I made a list of people to whom I needed to make amends (Step Eight). I had already made many of my amends as I wrote my inventory, but there was one I hadn't yet taken care of. When my sister and I were in grade school, we beat up two other girls on the way home from school. I was troubled because those girls had moved from our hometown long ago, and I knew of no way to contact them. My sponsor asked, "If you could, would you?" When I responded that I would, she advised me that willingness is sometimes good enough, that the requirement of Step Eight is simply that I be "willing to make amends to them all."

Through prayer and meditation (Step Eleven), I have come to rely on the God of my childhood. I was blocked from Him because of the food and because I didn't know how to access Him; my prayers had been like a wish list to Santa Claus. But any power that can remove my food obsession can do anything.

From time to time, when I try to solve my own problems (usually created through my selfishness and self-centeredness) instead of depending on Him, I begin to eat more. I begin to react to others and situations that I will not accept. I then have to decide whether I want to stay miserable or whether I will use the tools to try to reestablish conscious spiritual contact through working the Steps. Service (Step Twelve) is an important tool that I use to rid myself of the selfishness and self-centeredness that is the root of my problem. Shortly after I had given away my inventory, I volunteered to give service at an OA regional convention. I indicated on my registration that I would do whatever service was needed, but I wasn't thrilled when I received my confirmation with a request to be a hugger. So I did it a minute at a time for twenty-five minutes, greeting people and acting as if I loved it.

From the opposite direction came a very tall woman. I was pleased to notice she had been greeted—she already had a name tag on—and as she approached, I noticed her name. I only knew one other person with that name: the girl I'd beaten up in grade school. I asked her if I could speak with her, and I made my last amends. God really does for me what I cannot do for myself, if I get out of the way.

Through working the Steps, I discovered much pain surrounding the abuse from my father. He had died a few years before I came to OA, and I did much writing regarding our relationship. How I hated him. How I hated the fact that I was so much like him. I wrote him a letter and read it on his grave in the snow, but still I had no peace. Still I hated him. Still I resented that he didn't care for me as I wanted to be cared for.

After a lot more writing, giving it away, recognizing my part, and finally, finally, being willing to forgive him, I received peace. I heard a comforting voice tell me, "I am your Father and I have always loved you." I don't know whether that voice was my spiritual Father or my earthly father, but it doesn't matter. Today I can accept that it could have been both. Serenity only comes when I'm willing to let go and let God, through the Steps. Forgiving my father has made it possible to forgive myself and to ask forgiveness from my children. The ability to forgive came as a result of being open-minded about how he was raised and understanding that he was a product of the neglect and abuse of his childhood. The hope is that perhaps my children won't pass it on.

I have searched since childhood for someone to care for me. My parents didn't do it the way I wanted them to. My husband didn't do it the way I wanted him to. My sponsors and friends don't do it the way I want them to. I have learned that I am responsible for my own care. Since I released my husband from the responsibility, he has become very nurturing. In practicing the Third Step daily, I let God take care of me. When I do this, I am very, very well cared for, and I care for others. I possess what I searched for in food and in others. I have indeed experienced a personality change as the result of working the Steps. That change has made me become the person I always pretended to be. I am convinced it's elementary. I must live by the ABCs:

A. I am a compulsive overeater and cannot manage my own life;

B. Probably no human power—no husband, no children, no sponsor, no friend, no nutritionist, no doctor, no therapist, no weight-control center—could have relieved my compulsive overeating;

C. God can, and does, when He is sought.

7

Alive and Well and Living in the Real World

PRIOR TO MY INVOLVEMENT in Overeaters Anonymous, I never reacted normally to food, to other people, or to the events that occurred in my life. For most of my first thirty years, I remained separated from reality, as though I weren't connected to anything in this good world.

I was a stranger in my own family. I didn't realize it as a child, but my family provided me with nurturing and love, yet I was unable to accept it because of some twist in my personality that caused me to have unreasonable expectations of others. I have since come to believe that I was born with this defect, and that it had nothing to do with my environment or my family. I yearned to be like my two older brothers, yet I resented and secretly competed with them. If I couldn't win, I refused to play, even though my brothers were genuinely nice and gifted people. I probably was, too, but I was so absorbed in blaming others for the inadequacies of my life that I was unable to develop my own gifts. I declined to play a part in my own family. I was always at odds with them and with the world around me.

As early as kindergarten, I felt different from everyone. The girls I wanted for my friends were prettier than I—which meant they were not fat, and which also meant they were better than I. My other classmates were somehow lacking in my eyes. I saw everyone as a rival; I hid in the bushes during recess, wishing I could stay there alone forever. Food was the only companion I had.

One time, after receiving a spanking from my mother, I was so angry at her that I wished she would die. I felt furious but guilty for wishing such terrible things, and my insides were churning from crying. I went to the kitchen, ate a bologna sandwich, and immediately felt warm and comforted by the food. It made me feel everything would be all right. I've since learned that not everyone gets such comfort from eating a bologna sandwich, but food always made me feel good, and we were not in competition with each other.

During my high school and college years, I was the class clown, and I did have some friends by then. But I still felt as though I didn't really exist. Nothing mattered because I wasn't real. I believed that all the "real" girls had dates and bought pretty clothes and knew how to talk to people. I was fat, boring, and numb. To stay numb, though, I had to eat myself into oblivion.

During my second year at college, the pain of weighing 275 pounds at age seventeen became too painful, so I quit school and moved to another city. I had big plans for myself, big hopes that I could lose weight, start over, and change into a real person. It was all or nothing for me: either I was nobody or I was Miss America. I fantasized about moving away, losing weight, and returning to my campus thin and beautiful to break all the boys' hearts who had previously ignored me. The fantasies I had and my plans for revenge were the only threads of hope that kept me going.

I obtained a job at the city attorney's office and found that I enjoyed working and was an efficient secretary. The people in my office treated me with respect and listened to me, giving me a sense of self-confidence. I met a girl there who was overweight, and we decided to help each other lose weight. We went on a high-protein diet and both lost a hundred pounds. We spent a great deal of time on the phone with each other, and even though we were very different, we shared a love for food. This was the first time in my life that I had been successful at losing weight, and I was convinced that dieting was the answer. In retrospect, I now know that what worked for me was talking with another compulsive overeater and caring about someone else as much as I cared about myself.

After I lost that hundred pounds, I was sure that I would never be fat again. Since I was no longer obese, I believed that I could now have a real life. This, however, turned out to be only the beginning of a merry-go-round of dieting, weight-loss, and weight-gain. Over the next ten years, I lost and gained a hundred pounds twice more (in addition to countless periods of starting diets in the morning and breaking them before noon). It was also the start of trying to live a life without food, which sent me straight to alcohol, drugs, and sex to cope. I knew nothing about life beyond compulsion.

I acquainted myself with all the self-help books about diets and being fat that I could find. I knew about calories, exercise, and nutrition. I learned about self-esteem and psychology. But all this self-knowledge could not stop me from eating compulsively; once I began, I could not stop. No amount of will power was sufficient to stop me from eating when the craving arose. None of this knowledge quieted the raging discontent inside me. At times I didn't even know that I was regaining the weight. My only clue was the daunting awareness that I had no clothes that fit me.

By the time I was thirty years old, I weighed 300 pounds, and it appeared to me that I would remain obese for the rest of my life. I had no tolerance for others, especially pretty, thin women. The competition I had always felt with those around me was now accompanied by hate and resentment. I had married a man I didn't love, merely because he would have me. I didn't believe that a fat girl like me had any choice as to whom she could marry, and I thought being married and having children would make me feel normal. It didn't.

In the spring of 1979, my home and most of my hometown were destroyed by a tornado. That day became known as "Terrible Tuesday," and it changed all our lives forever. The entire town looked like a war zone, with every landmark completely demolished. After this disaster, my obsession with eating became as painful as being fat. I always wanted to be thin, but never wanted to stop eating the way I ate. However, after the tornado, I could not bear the destruction around me without eating constantly. I was seven months pregnant at the time, and my doctors warned me that I was hurting myself and my baby, but even that knowledge couldn't stop my eating. I went straight from the doctor's office to the nearest restaurant to stroke that ever-present desire in me with food. I don't know how my body withstood the pain, but I remained this way for another three years.

Then I was watching television one day and saw an ad for an Overeaters Anonymous workshop to be held in my town. For some reason I decided to go to it, and I remember being excited about it even though I had no information about the organization. I had already given up on every other diet club. I recall being the first person at the workshop and feeling annoyed that it didn't start on time. I felt very uncomfortable once the workshop began, but I thought the speakers were amazing. I had never heard anyone admit to being controlled by food as I was, nor had I ever heard anyone absolutely state that she had a good, loving relationship with God. Everyone I'd ever heard talk about God always dripped with insincerity and sweetness and spoke in a language I could not relate to at all. However, the speaker at the OA workshop certainly spoke my language, felt as I felt about food, and spoke with absolute credibility when she stated that God had relieved her food obsession. That day, I came to believe that God could do something about my eating, too, because He had helped that speaker. After all, she was just like me.

After the workshop, it took me eight months to get to an OA meeting. I badly wanted to find God alone and on my own terms, but it would not happen that way for me. I went to the parking lots of eight OA meetings without rousing enough courage to go inside. My fear was powerful, but the pain of overeating finally became so intense that I somehow managed to make it from my car into a meeting.

During my first meeting, I was obsessed that someone I knew would come in and see me there. To add to my irritation, only about nine people were there (all women), and one woman had on a dress just like mine. How dare she! My mind was in such turmoil that I couldn't even hear the words people were saying. God worked in my life that night, though, because at the end of the meeting I purchased a "Big Book," hoping to use it to recover and never have to go to another damned Overeaters Anonymous meeting. I've heard many people say they felt at home at their first OA meeting, knowing this is exactly where they belonged. Not so with me. Going to OA meant admitting I was fat, and I hated that truth more than anything else in my life—and believe me, I hated a great deal about myself and this world.

I started reading the "Big Book" at home, and in every instance where it used the word "alcohol," I crossed it out and put in the word "food." As I read this book, my life began to unfold in front of me. I cried and I laughed, because, for the first time, I understood so much. That night, while reading the "Big Book," I saw and heard what I'd denied about myself all my life. I could hardly wait for the next OA meeting, so I could ask the people there if they, too, grasped what this book said. I was on fire with excitement. At last I was real, and I was alive. That was 150 pounds ago, and my weight has not wavered more than 10 pounds in the almost ten years since.

I didn't know much about God when I started, and I welcomed the idea that I could entertain any conception of a Higher Power that I wanted to choose. I decided that if my ceiling were to fall on me, then it would be a power greater than myself, so I designated the ceiling in my bedroom my Higher Power. As I prayed to my ceiling, God began introducing Himself to me in very subtle ways. I diligently searched for Him as though he were a million dollars hidden in my living room. I watched TV preachers, joined a church, and went to open AA and OA meetings and conventions. I read AA's *Came to Believe*, and I read my "Big Book" every night. I offered myself to God as willing to do whatever it took to know Him better and to recover from this disease.

The answer proved to be completely spiritual. All I had to do was clean out the garbage of my past by working the Twelve Steps. God would do the rest. Cleaning house has been the basis of my recovery and my newfound relationship with God. I've put a great deal of time and effort into my prayer, inventories, and meditation. It is in my meditation that I have come to personally know God and feel His acceptance of me.

I'm sure that some of the things I've experienced while in His quiet presence could be rationalized as mere figments of my imagination, but I don't analyze and worry about such things anymore. I know how important my meditation has been to my emotional balance and healing. I also don't work too much on my emotional issues or worry about my weight. As the program says, when the spiritual malady is overcome, the emotional and physical recovery come naturally and easily.

I have made many mistakes during my recovery and have behaved quite badly at times. I have divorced, remarried, and divorced again. I still harbor such defects of character as jealousy, selfishness, and immaturity. My feelings still get hurt like a five-year-old child's; I sometimes sulk and plan my revenge. I have found, though, that as long as I keep trying, praying, and providing service in OA, God keeps me abstinent and doesn't judge me too harshly.

As a very judgmental person, this tolerance is something I would like to better give myself. At the end of our OA meetings, I ask God to forgive my trespasses—my shortcomings—as I forgive those who trespass against me. I stop and reflect on how forgiving I am of others. I can hold a grudge for a long time, but I've come to know that resentment paves the way for me to eat compulsively again.

I have a long way to go in my recovery, but my life is infinitely better than it was. I care about others, I perform service, and I belong in the OA Fellowship and in the world. I am happy for most of every day. I get along well with my family and have an active, productive life. The best part, though, is that I am no longer obsessed with food, and I no longer fight the fat. Today, I often say with a laugh that no matter what happens, it's a good day when I am abstinent and not married to my first husband. But in truth, I give all the credit for my recovery to God, whom I know personally. I have a great appreciation for how far our relationship has come from the days when I chose my ceiling as a Higher Power.

I would like to say something about the gift of sponsorship in this program. Some people think we should have sponsors more "advanced" than we are, but my sponsor and I came into Overeaters Anonymous at the same time. I have come to love her as I love no other human being. She knows absolutely everything about me, and the acceptance we give each other is a human reflection of God's love. We both have a great respect for the disease of compulsive overeating and the powerlessness that accompanies it. She encourages me and inspires me to want to live, to love, and to know God better, for she is goodness and love. Each day I thank God for this woman.

The benefits of living the spiritual life are immeasurable, and I am so thankful to be another of God's precious miracles.

8 ——————————

Alone No More

•

FOOD WAS ALWAYS the great pacifier for me. When I was a child, our family of five sat down to a dinner table stacked with a towering amount of food: five entire chuck steaks; mounds of potatoes, noodles, and rice. There was always more food than we could possibly have eaten. But night after night, my mother prepared it all. I looked forward to dinner each day as the only predictable love and security I knew.

I had regular nightmares when I was young. I remember seeing a pattern in the wallpaper one night that looked like a skull. In terror, I bolted into the kitchen and finished off a half gallon of fudge-marble ice cream. It was four in the morning, I was eight-and-a-half years old, and I'd found my way out of fear.

I shut myself off from friends and social gatherings, except when food was involved. I especially loved holiday gatherings because of all there was to eat. My personality changed when I ate. I became outgoing, aggressive, and opinionated. While I was usually scared of people, I now could argue with anyone, whether I knew what I was talking about or not.

As a teenager, my eating began to affect my health. I had gout, chest pains, high blood pressure, and frequent headaches. I weighed about two-hundred and fifty pounds at my draft physical, which I failed. The doctor told me that if I didn't lose weight, I'd be dead in a year. That got my attention, and I lost seventy pounds. Through college, though, I was an angry loner. I distrusted women; they were attracted to me now that I was thin and had been repulsed by me when I was fat.

A pattern of dieting and overeating began to emerge. I found diets on which I would lose a lot of weight. I maintained strict control for a while before returning to my old habits, ultimately reaching a higher weight than before I'd started.

I supported myself playing trumpet with a couple of local bands around Detroit. Because I cared about my stage appearance, I constantly pressured myself to look good; I was alternately fat and thin in these bands. It wasn't just how the obesity appeared that bothered me. It was my awkward, ill-at-ease stage presence that got in the way of my pretense of being a hip, slick, and cool entertainer.

When I met my former wife, I weighed 270 pounds. Our first dinner together was a chef's salad for her and chocolate doughnuts with coke for me. When we married in 1972, I was no more equipped for marital responsibility than a twelve-year-old. I picked fights, got sullen, fell over myself apologizing, became ravaged by guilt, and overate. Soon we became eating buddies. Years later, I came to Overeaters Anonymous because of the sickness of this relationship.

For years, I tried to build a career as a musician. I spent my days sleeping late, watching soap operas with a tremendous lunch, followed by a drink and a short nap. That one drink as dessert became two, then four, then six; I'd wake up sweaty and nauseous at five o'clock wondering where the day had gone.

My ex-wife had been an OA member, off and on, for quite a few years. She hadn't lost weight and she talked about God, so I concluded that she'd joined a cult for weak and simple-minded people. Of course, I was getting bigger by the day. But around this time, I became associated with a man who'd been sober in AA for about nine years.

It was through this man that I went to an OA meeting in 1979. I got there early, and I saw only women there. I immediately became defensive and refused to walk inside. Our friend met us there, and his response to my stubborn refusal to go into the meeting became very important in my eventual recovery.

"You can keep killing yourself if you want to," he said, "but I'm here to survive, like the other people in there. So what's it going to be?" He went inside without waiting for my answer. I was galled to be treated this way, but his words stuck. Yet I continued to become more fearful, angry, and withdrawn.

The height of my shame came when I had to buy a first-class seat on a plane because that was the only place I could fit. This humiliation played a big role in my eventual surrender.

What finally brought me to my knees—and to my senses— was an affair I had with my sister-in-law. I'd been alienated from my wife and felt very lonely in my marriage; my sister in-law colluded with me in an attitude of us against the world.

When my sister-in-law checked herself into a treatment center for alcoholism, I was devastated. The effects of carrying all these secrets around for six months had accumulated: I was having serious chest pains and could hardly breathe. When I went to a doctor, I discovered that I'd gained 75 pounds, not the 20 pounds that I'd expected. I again weighed 325.

I sat at the dining room table alone that night, not knowing what to do. I suddenly remembered the words I'd heard outside that OA meeting four years earlier. I called OA to see if there was a meeting that night. The truth was unavoidable: I couldn't stand myself or my life anymore. It was at two minutes before eight that evening that the last of my old life fell away.

A woman with three months of abstinence led the meeting that evening. I felt a warmth, caring, and acceptance in that room that I cannot recall ever experiencing. Not only did I belong there, but people wanted me there. My spiritual experience came when the leader looked me in the eye and asked me how I was doing. I said, "I never have to be alone again, do I?" I started to cry. I have been abstaining ever since that day over seven years ago and now maintain a weight loss of 150 pounds.

I felt three things in an overwhelming rush that night that I'd never felt before: trust, love, and willingness. Though I am an imperfect human being, often stumbling in my life, I have a heartfelt trust in God, a love for my fellows, and a willingness to live a life of principles, which allow me to abstain— no matter what.

Within the first week, I decided to throw every bit of my

mind and heart into understanding this program. My first Higher Power was the group. Atheist that I was, this was a big step. Then I became willing to accept the idea of a universal force, a cosmic order. It must have been quite amusing for the old-timers to listen to my arguments at ten days of abstinence about the existence of God. But even talking about God was a marvel; even that was evidence of a Higher Power working in my life. That Higher Power has enabled me to abstain, to change, to face who I am, and to take risks I never have taken before.

The holiday Yom Kippur occurred during my first week in the program. In the past, I'd either ignored it or fasted as a self-punishment, but this time it was different. I went to the synagogue and discovered that my religion and my OA program had a lot in common. Yom Kippur is a day set aside for inventory and amends. I prayed and reflected on my life, and for the first time, this holiday had meaning.

I was taught in OA that the action of love is service. I was told never to turn down an OA request for service, unless I was physically unable to perform it. I became a sponsor and an intergroup representative; I acted on the belief that I always have time to help another overeater. If I don't have time, I make time.

Of all the service positions I've held, my two favorites are acting as world service delegate and taking out the trash at my home meeting. I've found that I can handle a larger variety of responsibility than I'd thought. Most important, the food and weight just aren't problems anymore.

Overeaters Anonymous has given me a treasure chest of incredible experiences, along with the unshakable knowledge that I never have to be alone again, as long as I remember what

I used to be like and what I am like now. Thanks to all of you who have touched my life in the past, helped me enjoy the gift of the present, and given me an ever-growing hope for the future.

9

It Gets Better, I Promise

"MY NAME IS ROSE, and I am a compulsive overeater." I am so accustomed to uttering this phrase at meetings that I am hard-pressed not to use it whenever I introduce myself. Yet, even if I repeat it sometimes out of habit, it expresses the most significant facts about me: I am powerless over food, and a power greater than myself can restore me to sanity.

This disease took me to nearly three-hundred pounds on a small, five-foot-four-inch frame. I thank God there is a solution though; I have lived five and a half years at a healthy weight and, even more important, I am no longer a slave to food. I have always known I did not respond normally to food. I was also always overweight, increasingly so as the years progressed. When I was about ten, my doctor put me on a diet because, as he said, "You don't want all the other kids to call you 'fatty,' do you?" Did I want to be called names? Of course not. Could I, therefore, go on a diet? No. Nor could I explain this inability to anyone else. And so my loneliness began.

I started to diet at around age fifteen. Until I came into OA at age twenty-eight, I was either on a diet, pretending to be on a diet or planning to start a diet on Monday, the first of the month, or the first of the year. At the end of that thirteen-year period, I was about one-hundred pounds heavier than when I'd commenced the "diet era." That's what I call negative dieting.

My favorite of all my increasingly insane attempts to lose weight was what I now call the "new math diet." When I ate something, I'd assign it a very rough (and ridiculously low) calorie estimate. Then, of course, I'd want another, so I'd redo the math of what I'd already eaten to a lower calorie estimate. Ultimately, I lost progressively less weight each week, then stayed the same, then started gaining. I was sure other dieters were not so unfairly afflicted. It wasn't until I came to OA that I understood this anomaly—each week I ate more food!

The only time I felt carefree was when I postponed my diet to sometime in the distant future and gave myself free reign with the food. I carried around large bags of food, fantasizing my perfect life when I got thin—usually a cross between a *Leave It to Beaver* episode and the wedding scene from *The Sound of Music*.

I was certainly unhappy with my appearance, and I was bankrupt emotionally and spiritually, but it was the physical agony that brought me to OA. I was unable to walk and breathe comfortably. I couldn't find a comfortable sitting position. When I walked up the hill to my office, I was so out of breath, I couldn't speak. I had an obesity-related condition called sleep apnea that caused me to wake in the night choking for air. Claustrophobia closed in on me, a natural result of the extra 150 pounds sitting on my chest.

I even reached the point where I truly did not want to continue overeating, and still I could not stop. I ambled through stores in a supermarket-induced catatonia, unable to find anything to satisfy me. Even if I left the store empty handed, the food possessed me. (I never say food was my "drug of choice." I had no choice.) I had nightmares of being unable to lift myself off the bed. As I approached my twenty-eighth birthday, I'd all but given up hope. I knew I was dying.

It was during this period that I was given the answer before I even knew what the question was. My cousin, a grateful member of AA who lived in another town, Twelfth-Stepped me when I went to visit her. I went to an open AA meeting, and it was the greatest thing that ever happened to me.

When the speaker began, my cousin whispered, "Every time he says 'alcohol,' think 'food.'" I don't remember what he said, but I was in tears. I knew he was talking about me. But it wasn't the first Monday in January, so I couldn't start my annual diet. I had the most miserable two weeks of eating ever. On Sunday night, as I concluded the dreary business of the night before the diet, I felt relieved when I finished the last bit of junk food. I knew I couldn't stop until none was left.

There really is no way to adequately explain what happened next. The following day, I went to an OA meeting. By the grace of God, I have been abstinent ever since. The only thing I'd done to deserve it was to eat compulsively for twenty-eight years. I still don't understand it; grace is essentially a mystery. I know that God did for me what I could never have done for myself; I also know this gift is always available to me and to anyone else who wants it.

What I discovered in OA is that I have a disease. Compulsive eating is not a moral issue. I'm not a fool, nor am I weak-willed or a pig. I have a progressive disease. If I were to go back to overeating, it would be worse than before.

I also learned that I am a food addict. I am physically addicted to certain foods, as well as mentally addicted to all foods. In recovery, I cannot eat some foods at all, including sugar, flour, and most other high-carbohydrate items. No one told me which foods to stay away from; my sponsor suggested I pray for guidance, and this is the guidance I received.

It is critical that I talk to other OAers specifically about my food. I must keep vigilant, because my disease is extremely patient. As a friend of mine says, "You're either surrendering to God or you're surrendering to the food." Surrendering to food means death for me. I'm certain that I never have to eat compulsively again, but I will always be a compulsive overeater.

The loss of 150 pounds was both exhilarating and terrifying. At first I felt exposed if someone noticed my weight loss. But now I want strangers to applaud as I walk down the street. I want them to point and say, "Did you see that woman? She's a normal weight!" I discovered parts of me I didn't know I had. One night, I sat straight up in bed because I could feel my breast bone with each breath. I had to sit down with a friend and point out various bones that were new to me. "Do you have a bone there?" I asked. She assured me she did. Sometimes I take my body size for granted, but at times I look at myself in the mirror with a sense of awe and humility that something as close to me as a 150-pound weight loss was not my doing, but the work of a power greater than myself.

Maintaining my abstinence depends absolutely on the

Twelve Steps, as does the maintenance of my emotional and spiritual healing. I have had a great deal of growing up to do. My compulsion had arrested my normal maturing process, and I think I was emotionally around twelve years old when I came to the program. I think I'm up to twenty-one now!

Essentially, the Steps tell me to get out of myself and make contact with other people and with God. They direct me to look at my part in any troubling situations. When all I can see is someone else's wrongs, real or imagined, things only get worse. I came into this program paralyzed by extreme fears and resentments. Through the Steps, I no longer have to be ruled by these overwhelming moods. I've been blessed by a great sponsor and other comrades in the program who encourage me to turn inward and listen quietly for the voice of my Higher Power.

My Higher Power gives me the freedom from compulsive overeating and a way of living that absolutely works, even at the toughest times. I have had my share of pain in these five and a half years—primarily caused by the death of my parents two years apart. God's grace has given me abstinence and the ability to live in the present emotionally, without residual guilt. Grief has almost overwhelmed me, but God has helped me cope with it.

My grandiose *Sound of Music* plans have not panned out, but I have received things it never occurred to me to dream for: real peace of mind, true love, and contentment in my heart. My sponsor had often said to me in the midst of my despair, "It gets better. I promise." I believed her, and it has gotten better and better and better. Just keep coming back through the despair, and it can get better for you, too.

10

Growing Up in OA

       I CAME INTO OA shortly after I turned fifteen years old. I have spent my formative years in OA; consequently, I've been able to experience many critical events in my life that I would have otherwise been too depressed to notice.

I've been a compulsive overeater since birth. I wondered as early as nursery school why any other child would want to be my friend, since I thought of myself as fat and ugly. When I entered elementary school, I alienated myself from my classmates. My world consisted of going to school, watching TV, snacking, eating dinner, and then sneaking food all evening. I didn't leave the house except to buy ice cream or candy.

My grandfather, who'd been my only friend, died when I was eight years old. My world fell apart. I stopped believing in God and wanted to commit suicide, yet I was terrified of dying. My parents said I was too young to be depressed; that was the last time I told them how I felt.

My weight kept creeping up. Food was my joy and my escape. My parents made me participate in social activities, such as the Boy Scouts, which I only tolerated because of the refreshments. I had to eat a little bit all the time. When I went to summer camp, I stole money and bought as much candy as possible to get me through the week. I told people I loved food. The truth was that I never enjoyed eating because I was always thinking about the next thing I would eat.

Until I was ten, I didn't associate my love for food with my weight problem. I thought I'd been born fat and that fat was simply my destiny. But my father took me on a trip to Israel when I was ten to visit relatives; this was the first time I was away from my mother, with whom I did a lot of secret eating. I was out of my environment and didn't have a chance to think about the food. I lost fifteen pounds, which everyone noticed, and I realized for the first time that I might be able to control my weight. I still felt fat, but everyone told me how good I looked. Since at the time I was already wearing adult sizes, I decided to start dieting.

Every Sunday night I ate as much as I could, because Mondays meant the start of the strictest diet I could find. I felt I should eat nothing because I was so fat. I thought I might go crazy from boredom and depression, so the diets only lasted a day or two. I'd eat one extra bite of something so I could say I'd blown it and eat anything I wanted. By the time I was twelve years old, I was seventy pounds overweight, and my doctor told my parents that I'd weigh 250 pounds by the time I graduated from high school.

When I was about to enter junior high school, my mother (my binge buddy) went to OA. She forced me to go to a few meetings with her; I thought OA might be good for her, but I was too young. My mother thrust her food plan on the rest of us, leaving me scavenging the cupboards in the evenings while she went to meetings. I even binged on salads. I convinced myself that I would "outgrow" my obesity.

My junior-high years were misery. I was placed in a special physical education class, where I had to jog around the track every day. I was the slowest one. I thought I was having a heart attack every day, and it felt that the whole world was looking at me and laughing. I felt like dying every time I had to change my clothes in the locker room. I was almost friendless.

During the summer before entering high school, my mother got involved in OA again, and she asked me to go to a meeting with a friend's son. I don't know why I agreed to it, but I went. There were six teens and one adult leader. It wasn't like my Mom's meetings; everyone just talked. I couldn't see how all this talking had anything to do with weight, so I didn't participate. I just looked forward to starting school, when I hoped I would be unable to eat all day.

When I started school that fall, I felt that OA was my last chance. I asked the people at my meeting if they had suggestions that might stop my daily purchase of cookies and candy from the student store. They recommended that I call and commit what I would eat for the day to another OA member. It sounded logical to me. But the food I was committing to was not diet food, so I didn't think it was abstinence. I lost weight, though, despite good-sized meals. This surprised me and made me aware of how much I'd been eating. Although I felt better, I wasn't interested in any other part of OA.

I started another teen meeting, which got me involved in other meetings and the intergroup as a way to publicize this group. I was on an OA high. I lost twenty-five pounds, became taller, and began to make friends. I felt alive for the first time. I even started to go to parties and talk to girls, which had once seemed impossible.

I heard my OA friends talk about miracles and God, and it finally dawned on me that a power had touched my life. I asked our group leader to be my sponsor, and he directed me to begin a Fourth-Step inventory. I thought I would never have the courage to write down all my secrets and complete an inventory. My sponsor said that I had to take responsibility for my life and quit blaming my parents for my misery, or I would surely go back to the food. I read my inventory to my sponsor, who then helped me work on my amends and character defects. I felt a deep sense of peace.

When I graduated from high school in 1979, I was a normal weight (not the 250 pounds my doctor had predicted), and I couldn't believe I'd lived that long. I was grateful to hear the stories of older OAers who'd missed out on such events of their youth as their high school prom. I'd gone to my prom, participated in my graduation, and felt that I was available to that part of my life because of OA.

I started college in the fall, even though I thought I was stupid, because I knew my OA friends would still be there if I failed. I eventually received a degree in accounting because I was willing to balance the demands of work and school along with my OA program. I would never have survived college if I'd been into the food. Many times I was lonely and broke, but I kept my abstinence and commitment to the program.

What was once a terrible relationship with my parents has been healed beyond belief through these sixteen years in the program. I do service for my family as I do in OA. I've also been in a relationship with a woman in OA for the past several years. I never thought I could manage the daily ups and downs of an intimate relationship, but we share a real joy. We've traveled together, which has shown me that God and a flexible abstinence can be taken all over the world.

Sixteen years later, I still go to at least one OA meeting per week. Usually food is not a problem, but I am grateful for the times that the obsession takes over because it reminds me that I still need to grow in OA.

One of the keys to my long-term abstinence has been to stay active in OA service. It helps me stay connected to my past and to cherish the miracles that happen when we reach out to one another. Service keeps me from becoming complacent, and I'm certain that whatever help I give to OA can never repay the help OA has given me.

Physically, OA has helped me maintain a normal weight for the past fifteen years. Spiritually, OA has helped me see that I'm not in charge of this world. I trust in a Higher Power and no longer am paralyzed when I have to make a decision. Emotionally, OA has helped me to love myself. I have confidence and feel like a worthy human being. I can walk with my head up and can even live with tragedy without eating over it.

Today, my life is more exciting than ever. I used to think that if I worked the program and eliminated all the self-imposed negativity from my life, I'd get bored. Sometimes I think there are no miracles left to experience or achievements for me to reach for, but I'm always wrong. Life doesn't stop changing and, for today, I'm not so afraid of dying because I've learned to live!

11

New Hope at Age Sixty

ONE OF MY EARLY memories concerns my father sending my brother to bed without his supper. To deprive a hungry child of a meal was unforgivable in my mind, since we children worked hard at our chores on the farm after school. I promised myself then that I would never let this happen to me. I would always find food somewhere. It was puzzling to me that my brother did not grab and gulp the food I sneaked up to him later on, but simply turned in his bed and cried himself to sleep. At this early age, food deprivation seemed intolerable to me.

At thirteen, I left home to enter a convent preparatory school in Milwaukee, some eight-hundred miles from my rural Nebraska home. Visiting day was the second Sunday of the month. I was too far from home to have visitors, but I still delighted in the goodies my classmates' visiting relatives brought them. I often felt ashamed of how much of their sweets I hid, saved, and consumed for comfort in my lonely hours.

I was a tall, strong, rural kid, so I was often assigned duties requiring muscle alongside the older girls. We were generally rewarded for our heavy lifting and cleaning jobs with tasty snacks or lunches. Needless to say, I was flattered to be part of any job that paid in hot chocolate and cookies.

Strangely, my preoccupation with food did not put extra weight on my body for many years. But my addiction expressed itself during nearly thirty years of convent life in celebrating every special day with a banquet—whether a birthday, saint's day, holiday, or just plain Sunday. And feast I did! Usually the table or food preparation was my focus of criticism. I am deeply chagrined, even now, to recall that my external life was one of discipline and renunciation, while food and meals were actually my greatest focus. Because of the regularity of my convent and teaching routine, random eating was not prevalent, but I did salvage food left in children's abandoned lunch bags to use for my secret predinner feasts. During all those years, I felt gluttonous, guilty, and embarrassed over my misuse of food.

I entered graduate school in the summer of 1969 and roomed with other students who were nuns. We shared a kitchen and the cooking. During the next three semesters we behaved like children just released from parental restraint. We competed to see who could come up with the richest, most novel dishes. We went crazy on cooking, eating, and studying, and I gained forty-five pounds. I was so steeped in the adventure of having a social life and eating at every available moment that I hardly noticed.

I was forty-five years old now, and the dieting finally

began. Newspaper ads, diet books, and weight-loss devices were suddenly my feverish pursuit. After graduation, and at my new teaching assignment, I carefully calculated how to obtain diet pills, replenish my wardrobe, and lie about my bloated body.

One day in 1972, a sixth-grade student stopped in my office, proud to tell me she was in a weight-loss program. She left a flyer on my desk. I found a local meeting site. Because I was a nun, I was offered a scholarship if I permitted the use of my picture for before-and-after weight-loss ads. Going from 196 pounds in October to 156 pounds in April made me eligible for their advertisements. As you can imagine, their value was short-lived for me.

The fifteen years between my forty-fifth and sixtieth birthdays were rich with important decisions and changes, but I was haunted by the strangling pain of the food compulsion. During these years I left the religious order, obtained a good job at a midwestern university, and married. Marriage was wonderful, and work was challenging, but neither of them contributed satisfactorily to my inner self-esteem. I simply did not know how to behave when food was available. My hidden eating increased, grazing became a habit, and my dishonesty about my weight, size, diets, and recipes grew. After many unpleasant episodes, I admonished myself with degrading thoughts about "this smart, capable woman who is a glutton!"

With our move to San Diego in 1978, I exchanged my teaching career for work in a psychologist's office. Ironically, I grew more and more insane in that therapeutic atmosphere, using food as a cure-all for any unpleasant or surprising emotions. I deeply resented my employer and workplace. My mood swings became so unpredictable that I sometimes hid from myself in the bathroom or a corner of the office. But I could be comforted, I thought, with just another doughnut, just one more sweet roll, and on and on. This behavior accompanied one last search for the ONE thing wrong with me; I was confident I could easily change, should I discover it. I consulted self-help books, sought out an allergist and an acupuncturist, wore an ear device, and dieted until both my energy and my purse were depleted.

During this period, I was doing volunteer work at a nonprofit bookstore and library on my days off. This center was two doors west of the main OA meeting center in San Diego. I criticized the members' manners and dress, as well as the language I overheard during their breaks. But the desperation following a Thanksgiving binge in 1984 drove me into the OA room early one Saturday morning.

I was a slow convert who resisted hugs, found fault with members, and surely was not one of "them." But I could not resist coming back, although I often left meetings angry and despondent. One day the ice thawed. Someone shared her pain-filled experience, and my heart broke with compassion. I hugged her warmly, and my OA life began in earnest. It was March 1985. New hope burned in my soul; I attended more meetings and found a sponsor. With her help, I soon realized OA is a movement, a progression, a step-by-step procedure that can pervade my life—not just my table, my refrigerator, and my grocery shopping.

Buried beneath the pounds—now 220 plus—was a deep longing for serenity, even more than for thinness. I was spiritually and psychologically exhausted from my lack of boundaries and my easily triggered mood swings. Slowly it dawned on me through Steps One, Two, and Three that the burden of my weight was intimately tied to the burden of my soul, and that abstinence from extra food was directly related to abstinence from stored-up resentments, self pity, and judgments.

A new world opened before me. I humbly followed a plan of double abstinence, from both excess food and excess brooding. My body forfeited fifty pounds, while my soul surrendered control and disdain. I found it critical to first accept my situation, then surrender to a Higher Power as I walked through Steps Four through Nine.

My sponsor's suggestions became a bit nebulous after Step Five. I feared I was now on my own until I heard about the importance of Step-study meetings. Since there were none in my immediate area, two seasoned OA members and I opened an afternoon Step study in a local library. At the organizational meeting, I learned the dynamics of group conscience, group service, and group anonymity, and that the method of study agreed upon was for everyone's spiritual benefit.

At these meetings, I saw living examples of serenity and self-esteem. I became physically and emotionally quieted; I was spiritually strengthened. Then, with confidence, I wrote to, called, and personally approached with my amends those that I had harmed. It was as though I were meeting these people for the first time. They were and are beautiful people! I wrote even to those who were deceased, with no excuses or explanations, only love.

My euphoria at this stage challenged my abstinence, and I gained five or ten pounds. I wanted to graduate and become the service person of all service people. I wanted to be done with the Steps. I was forgetting that Steps Ten and Eleven require daily attention and that Step Twelve has no timetable. At my sponsor's suggestion, I recorded what I ate each evening and graded each meal as moderate, high-moderate or compulsive. I continued this practice for a year. It resulted in a very detached feeling from the food compulsion.

My daily inventory often left me with a sense of failure because I was listing daily defeats. Each evening I was a sinner, until an intuitive inspiration came from page 550 in the "Big Book" explaining honesty, open-mindedness, and willingness. I chose to note the positive ways I had practiced these qualities during the day. Then I prayed and fell into a restful sleep. My shortcomings appeared gently in my morning meditations, in my writings, and in conversations with a sponsor or sponsorees.

More than that, I began to get a better sense of my place in the universe. I am here to love; I am here to learn; I am here to reestablish harmony. This is impossible to do in isolation, in withdrawal, or in egocentrism. But it is possible, one day at a time, if I stay in touch with my Higher Power in prayer and with my fellow OAers at meetings.

Sometimes, when I stand before a group at meetings to share, I am moved by the love and openness in the faces of my fellow compulsive eaters. I ask myself, "Where else could I recover, in the truest sense of the word, with so many others trying to improve their lives spiritually, emotionally, and physically?" I believe these efforts are the highest form of service to humankind, for love surely sends out vibrations and resonates in the waiting heart. At age sixty, a new day and a new hope dawned for me. I trust I'll be good for many more years of spreading OA's good news.

12

Deep Denial

"MY NAME IS RICHARD, and I'm a compulsive overeater in deep denial." That was how I introduced myself at my first OA meeting. I was six days sober, and the meeting had been "suggested" by a counselor from my treatment center. I was trying to be clever and defiant; I did not want to be there. Yes, I had been beaten by alcohol, I thought, but now that I'd stopped consuming all those alcoholic calories, my weight should go down.

But I conveniently overlooked some things. I forgot that my first drink was at age twenty-one, and my first diet was at age eight. It slipped my mind that I had been on and off diets and up and down the scale all my life. I didn't notice that I, morbidly obese at 349 pounds, was the only person out of the forty people in treatment who was sent to an OA meeting. How ironic that my very first statement in OA was the exact truth.

When it came to food, I was a garden-variety grazer and

general overeater. I had no concept of the difference between the food I needed and the food I wanted. It was all the same. If there was food, I wanted it. If I wanted it, I needed it, so I ate it. Sure, there were binges, but constant eating worked best for me.

I was uncomfortable with my eating and felt that other people were watching and judging me any time I ate. I tried to eat normally in front of other people, but I came back for more when no one was around. I would buy too much, cook it, eat it all, and hide the wrappers at the bottom of the garbage can. Or I might buy different varieties of fast food, acting as if I were trying to remember what other people had asked me to pick up for them.

When I had guests, I filled the plates in the kitchen. I ate quite a lot of the food before any got to the table. Then, of course, there was cleanup. Why throw perfectly good food in the garbage? I was puzzled at the special shame some people expressed at meetings over eating out of the garbage. It was automatic for me to dust the food off and eat it.

I am a compulsive feeder, as well. I remember hearing years ago that the sincerest form of affection is sharing food with another person. When I hosted a dinner party, I went all out. I put a great deal of energy and emotion into food preparation. The first year we had the family Thanksgiving at our house, I started planning in January; every month when my food magazine arrived, I started selecting recipes and testing them. We served a nine-course dinner for fourteen people. After all that, the food didn't get nearly the attention I thought it deserved. I was very disappointed. Didn't they realize how much love I was showing them? What was wrong to make them reject me this way? I was always depressed after one of these occasions, but I kept trying.

For the first five months in OA, I went to one meeting a week. Things were fine, and I was losing weight nicely. Then came that first Christmas. I went through three weeks of old-fashioned, holiday eating. This time I could see how little I really enjoyed the eating and how out of control I was around food. The OA message had sunk in just enough. After New Year's Day (a traditional day to clean up my act), I did it a little differently than in previous years. I started going to an OA meeting every day with the idea of attending ninety meetings in ninety days. I still go to some sort of Twelve-Step meeting six or seven times a week.

I didn't volunteer to take the Steps. My sponsor and his sponsor had organized a closed, committed Step study at my sponsor's house. I wasn't wild about this idea, but as a confirmed people pleaser, I had to go. I'm grateful now that I did. It kept me moving through the Steps.

It was the Fifth Step that impacted me most profoundly and immediately. Over a few hours, my whole attitude and outlook upon life and the people closest to me—particularly my wife—changed dramatically.

I read over what I had written as I waited on a bench by the beach for my sponsor. My sponsor had suggested using the format in the "Big Book," so each item was short. I thought about each resentment, each fear, each hurt. There it was. Not nice, nothing to be proud of, actually pretty dull. Was it enough? What would my sponsor think of me?

When he arrived, we began. As I went back through the items, sharing and expanding on them, I relived them one last time. I almost forgot about the ocean and my sponsor until I was done. My sponsor hugged me and told me he loved me. As

I started home, it didn't seem as if anything had changed.

When I got home, my wife was seated at the piano. I realized that the things about her that made me so angry and unhappy were no longer relevant. Some of the resentments were twenty years old! They just didn't matter anymore. I put my arms around her and started crying. It is an interesting coincidence that I have been abstinent since that day. This change in me is part of the reason my wife decided to join OA.

I had trouble with the idea of abstinence at first. I was cynical and judgmental and thought that abstinence was just another word for diet. "All right," I thought, "I'll play their little word games." When someone said her abstinence was not perfect, to me she was saying she wasn't abstinent, but took credit for it anyway. This attitude was part of the reason that I didn't maintain continuous abstinence. I was very exacting and set standards for myself that I couldn't possibly live up to.

Today, my abstinence is not perfect. If I were perfectly abstinent I would eat exactly what God wants me to eat, and I would feel absolutely no guilt or shame about eating it. Today, my Higher Power no longer expects that kind of performance from me and, best of all, I don't expect it from myself, either. When I pray, "Give us this day our daily bread," I am praying for my abstinence. Having asked God's help, I leave it up to Him.

I accept this body that God gave me and that it needs a certain amount of food. It was my self-will that added the extra food necessary to maintain my obesity. If I eat as God intended, I will have an average-sized body. Long before reaching my goal weight, I became a maintainer. I stopped trying to lose weight and started eating as if I had magically lost all the weight I needed to. I had learned the difference between being abstinent and being on a diet.

All was well for a few months. Then, after losing 115 pounds, the weight loss stopped. I accepted this for a month or so, but soon lost patience with God. I was still 35 pounds from the weight I had chosen as ideal for myself when I started. It would have been a nice, round (and very impressive, I thought), 150-pound weight loss.

I resolved to go back to dieting to lose those last few, stubborn pounds. To be very precise and scientific about it, I went to a hospital and had my body fat measured. I wanted to know exactly what was the right weight for me.

The results? I was at 18 percent body fat, right in the normal 10-20 percent range. The weight I had picked was an unreasonable 3½ percent, probably not even possible to achieve. God knew what He was doing after all.

I have been married nearly thirty years, and in that time my wife and I have thoroughly tested our marriage vows. Rich, poor, sick, healthy: Each of us has been to the brink of death due to our diseases. We stayed together through inertia and the mutual wish to avoid conflict at any cost, and we stayed together because it was in God's plan for us. I am very grateful that God kept us together, because now we are able to support each other's recovery. Our relationship is recovering, too, and we are creating a happy marriage.

One of the things we do together each day is a formal Tenth and Eleventh Step. We review our food and how we feel about it. We go over the day's activities, looking at both the good and bad aspects of the day. We always have a gratitude list with at least one item each. We feel there is always something to be grateful for in the day if we've paid attention at all.

I started out thinking that I could use only very special

incidents on this gratitude list: one of those rare flashes of deep thankfulness in the day. Now I try to include some of the ordinary things I normally take for granted. This must be what is meant by an "attitude of gratitude." I'm certainly grateful to be developing it.

We end our time together with our own little prayer. "God, let me know what your will is for me and for us as a couple, and give us the power to carry that out." It's a very nice way to end the day.

When I started the OA program, I said that I didn't believe in God. That was not true. When I was a child I suffered nightmares about going to hell. God, as I understood Him, had condemned me to hell for what I had done and hadn't done, what I had thought or hadn't thought. From an early age, I had hidden from God by pretending that He didn't exist.

The "Big Book" brought me out of hiding and showed me that maybe God did love me. At many meetings we read "How It Works," ending with the ABCs of the program. The last line, "God could and would if he were sought," caught my attention right away. God could do anything all right, but it never occurred to me that He would.

I have taken service positions all along in OA, not from any sense that it was important to my recovery, but more so that I would have a place in this Fellowship. My hand went up at every opportunity. I soon found myself with one or more service positions in each of the meetings I attended regularly.

Now I have only two service positions: one at the group level and one at the intergroup level. It is important that I limit my service positions for a couple of reasons. First, I belong at OA meetings simply because I don't want to eat compulsively. Second, I may be depriving another OA member of using one of the tools of the program.

I go to meetings these days because I want to, not because I need to. Desperation is rare for me and doesn't last long. I won't say that I never have thoughts about eating when I don't need to. The difference is that these thoughts don't dominate my mind as they used to. Usually, when I review the day, I find that I have not seriously considered eating between meals.

This year, I changed cities, started a new job, suffered a death in my immediate family, and said good-bye to both my children as they left to start their own homes. Being active in OA allows me to accept the things I cannot change, gives me the courage to change the things I can, and provides me the wisdom to know the difference. With God's help, I am peaceful, joyous, and comfortable with myself. Now that's what I call living!

13

Saying Yes to Life

WHEN I FIRST CAME to Overeaters Anonymous sixteen years ago, I was panic-stricken about my inability to diet and my mounting weight. Years earlier, I'd only needed to lose about twenty pounds, then it was forty pounds. By the time I got to OA, I was carrying an extra seventy pounds. I was terrified of exceeding 200 pounds, but at 195 and eating uncontrollably, I knew there would be no limit to my self-destruction.

I was raised by alcoholic parents and then married an alcoholic, so I could see the similarities between my eating and their drinking. I even called myself a "food-aholic." When I heard of OA, I felt a small hint of hope. My father had attended AA for a short time in 1966, and I had some familiarity with AA's success with alcoholics. But it wasn't easy to find a meeting in my area; there was no intergroup, meeting schedule, or phone line. I eventually found a Wednesday night meeting and attended.

In the past, I'd always persuaded friends to go to weight-loss groups with me. But for some reason—I suspect it was desperation—I attended my first OA meeting alone. It's hard to describe how moved I was to hear the stories of others who had used food as I did. They'd eaten it half-frozen; they'd burned their mouths because they couldn't wait for the food to cool; they'd sworn off overeating and then binged; they'd thrown food in the garbage and then dug it out to devour later.

For the first time, I knew I had a disease. At age thirty-two, I discovered I wasn't an awful failure and that others suffered as I did. And I had a name for it: compulsive overeating. A great load was taken from my shoulders. It was the first of many spiritual awakenings in OA.

I was on the verge of tears after the meeting. Embarrassed by my reaction, I wanted to run out after the closing prayer, but a woman who was to become my first sponsor gave me a hug and told me she could see I was in pain. I wept as she spoke to me. This was my first experience of one overeater reaching out to another, and I left the meeting hopeful that there might be a way out of my prison.

I've heard members say that OA has ruined their eating. I agree with that and would take it one step further. My life could never be the same after immersing myself in this program. I am no longer a victim. I take risks and dare to make mistakes. All this is a direct result of applying the Twelve Steps and OA's tools to all of my life, not just my eating.

Yet, I've struggled over the years with defining a plan of eating I could live with—a flexible, but effective, way of eating that is healthy and right for my body and that also allows me to enjoy eating. My old attempts at controlling my compulsive overeating involved long periods of deprivation that inevitably led to relapse. I was either dieting or bingeing.

Even though I struggled, I lost fifty pounds during my first few years in the program. I began to see, though, that the harder I tried to "put the plug in the jug" of my overeating, the more I seemed to fail. I was using OA as a diet club, forgetting that diet clubs had never worked for me before.

I talked with a woman in OA whom I admired. She helped me see that I was striving for a "perfect" abstinence with food, and that perhaps that was an unrealistic expectation. It was difficult to let go of my dream of perfection, but I found that once I was able to let go of those rigid requirements, the food called to me less and less. I began to accept myself as an imperfect human being.

Food was now less important, and I began to work the Steps with a sponsor and work with our intergroup. As I began to have more clarity, I could see many problems in my marriage that I'd been avoiding with food. I felt demoralized and desperate to have such serious doubts about my marriage. I relapsed again and thought of leaving the program for good.

At one Monday night meeting, a member brought a copy of *For Today* and read an excerpt from January 31 that encourages us to say yes to life. It was just what I needed to hear. Fear had been keeping me stuck in using food to handle my problems and prevented a deeper commitment to God. I got on my knees at home that night and vowed to say yes to life, in whatever form that might take. I took the Third Step in a more profound way than I had in the previous six years.

It has been my experience that my darkest moments usually come before a major surrender. When my self-induced pain becomes greater than my fear of the next Step, I become willing to take a leap. I am learning to envision my Higher Power as a safety net that is there for me when I decide to take the leap of faith.

My marriage eventually ended. Soon thereafter, my grandmother and father died. The love of the Fellowship carried me through and helped me maintain belief in a God that is always here for me, even when I can't feel the connection.

A few years later, a committee called the Twelfth Step Within was formed to help OA members in relapse. This committee gave my program a new focus of sharing my experience with those in our Fellowship who were suffering as I once had. This committee spoke to me as no previous movement in OA had. It addressed relapse as not only physical, but also emotional and spiritual. I began to hear that, for many of us, relapse was a part of our recovery. We could recover from relapse, not by beating ourselves up with the program, but by loving ourselves, showing up for meetings, and doing service.

Today my recovery includes no dieting. I no longer choose to suffer the highs of losing weight and the lows of failing yet again. I find myself with an attitude of joy and acceptance of myself as a human being with assets and defects. I know now that only God has control of my eating. I am truly powerless.

One thing has remained constant over these turbulent years: my commitment to recovery in the OA program. My goal is to follow the principles of this program and to stay out of my Higher Power's way. I am committed to daily prayer and meditation, attending OA meetings, providing service, and working the Twelve Steps in all areas of my life.

Today I say yes to life. Just as our disease takes many different paths before we come together in OA, so does our recovery once we are here. This is the message I carry: No matter what, just keep coming back!

14

The Graveyard Shift

My childhood is a blur, but I remember my teen years well. I was fat and uncoordinated, and I developed large breasts. The small church where I played piano for services was my only escape from my peers' name calling and my own shame. I decided to make a career in the church as either a musician or administrator and could hardly wait to get out of high school and into Bible college.

But I quickly learned that the church is not exempt from discrimination against the obese. I auditioned for our denomination's choir. I had assumed I would be chosen, so when the rejection letter arrived, I wondered if I'd been turned down because of my appearance. One of my music teachers said that my voice was very good, confirming my suspicions that my obesity had been the deciding factor. The lives of teenagers can be rough enough as they try to find their place in the world, but for a fat young man with pimples and low self-esteem, the future is very intimidating.

My father told me to get a job. I saw a listing in the paper for a graveyard-shift hotel clerk that seemed inviting to me. To work while the rest of the world slept seemed ideal. They hired me, and my self-imposed isolation was set in motion.

I raided the hotel kitchen at night without interruption. I had my food and was removed from external criticism. I thought I was set for life. As I continued to gain weight, I was turned down for similar graveyard-shift positions because of my size; I lost one job because I failed the physical. The doctor told me my high blood pressure from obesity would kill me before I was thirty. I felt I had no reason to live anyway.

Early on, I decided to live just for today—years before the program's motto became a way of life—but I could never get enough food. I ate out of grocery bags on my way home from the store and had my meals from serving bowls so I wouldn't have to get up to serve myself again. I wish I could say this is exaggerated, but it is painfully true. It only ended as I collapsed into bed each night. The routine continued for years.

Each resolve to diet ended back in the old habits. Twice I lost one-hundred pounds, only to gain it back in half the time it took to lose it. I seemed fated to a life of overeating and obesity. Then the food turned on me. I began to have pains in my left arm and chest, and I had to prop myself up in bed to be able to breathe. I was scared of dying, and the food was losing its appeal. I didn't enjoy it but was compelled to keep eating. Every day I vowed to change, but I could not stop. I was like a drug addict: I had to have it. There was no joy, just a fix.

One Sunday morning I went to church instead of to the grocery store. I was uncomfortable in my too-tight clothes—I wore a tie to hide the gaps in my dress shirt—and church itself was disappointing, but it kept me out of the food. Even though I reverted to my serving-bowl supper the next day, my recovery began that Sunday.

I took more action, joining a weight-reduction program that sells prepackaged food. They wanted to weigh me, but their scales only went to 450 pounds. I went to a local hospital where I weighed in at 458. I attended behavior-modification classes, but could hardly fit into the desk, which made listening difficult. All I could think of was getting out of there without taking the desk with me. For two weeks, I ate their food and listened to their tapes, and it was hell. In the third week, I ordered a pizza and fell into the immediate depression of failure. Why couldn't I control my food like other people? There appeared to be no hope.

At least ten years earlier, someone had mentioned Overeaters Anonymous to me. I was rude to him when he tried to tell me about his weight loss, but I never forgot that he'd been helped in OA. Now I was desperate; my own best efforts had failed.

I couldn't admit to being a compulsive overeater at my first meeting, but I decided to keep coming back. I always arrived early to find a comfortable chair and left as soon as we said amen. I bought all the literature, though, and it was through the literature that I discovered the program.

The meetings confused me. Most of those who came didn't appear to have a problem; they weren't morbidly obese. Once I spoke to someone at a meeting who'd talked of difficulty she was having with a certain food. Why shouldn't she just eat it, I asked, since it wasn't showing up on her body? The leader lovingly corrected me, explaining that our disease cannot always be detected by body size, and that bulimics and anorexics were also members of our group. He also advised that I not engage in crosstalk or offer advice during the meeting. I had a lot to learn, but they were patient with me.

I noticed that the most solid aspect of the program seemed to be the Twelve Steps, so I started taking them. I assumed it wouldn't take long; reading through them seemed simple enough.

I learned I was to have a sponsor. That seemed impossible to me because I had such low self-esteem I could not ask anyone for help. I called the intergroup office and explained to the gentleman answering the phone what a special case I was, since I weighed over four-hundred and fifty pounds. I am sure he chuckled to himself as he explained that he'd lost two-hundred fifty pounds in OA. I asked him if it was possible to lose the weight without a sponsor. He told me there are no rules in OA, but that people who recover do have sponsors. It seemed safe enough to ask over the phone if I could call him for the next ten days. He didn't say no! Ten days passed, and I kept calling.

I began to lose weight on what I now consider to be three binges a day. Even with those flexible guidelines, I broke my abstinence the third week and was engulfed with the old sense of failure. I called my sponsor to tell him the program had not worked for me. He asked me what I usually did when I went off my diets. Well, I continued to eat, of course! He reassured me that I was in recovery because I had called him instead of continuing to overeat. These were important words for me to hear. I learned an important tool that day: Tell it, get rid of it, and move on with your life.

I finally agreed to meet with this person who was becoming a friend over the phone. He shared with me his method for working the Fourth Step, so I proceeded as he suggested. I was full of fear about the Fourth Step, since it was followed so closely by the Fifth; I couldn't imagine revealing all the depraved aspects of myself to anyone.

To help me through this fear, he suggested I write down the things I thought I could reveal and on a second sheet all the things I might be able to reveal in the future. On a third sheet, I was to write down what I would never be able to tell anyone. I completed the Fourth Step in a few weeks, and when it came time to do the Fifth Step, I was ready to get rid of it all. I was ready to challenge the program to see if it worked. It was, of course, a wonderful experience. My sponsor knows me better than anyone else, and I'm able to share myself honestly with him today.

I now realize we don't "work" the Twelve Steps. It is a continuing process of taking inventory, seeking a relationship with a power greater than ourselves, and sincerely trying to carry the program to those who still suffer. Today I am living free from the bondage of the old routine I could not escape on my own. I have lost 237 pounds and can wear jeans with a T-shirt tucked in for the first time in my life. I cannot take credit for these results. It was through the Steps that God restored me to sanity. My Higher Power continues to work in and through me, if I remain willing to remember who I am and who God is.

I'm still working the graveyard shift, but I'm not hiding anymore. I have bad nights and good nights, but I accept—with support—whatever life hands me. Life is just beginning for me, and the graveyard is not my goal.

15 _____

Losing Pounds, Gaining Ground

I BELIEVE I WAS born a compulsive overeater. When I was eighteen months old, my parents found me on the floor, sharing a bone with our labrador retriever. At age three, I discovered "trick or treating": the next time Mom wouldn't give me candy, off I went to the neighbors. It worked once, why not again? I started manipulating people and circumstances early in life to get more food.

This was the beginning of a lifetime centered on food and weight. I felt inadequate and flawed and was terribly self-conscious about my appearance. At age six, when my dance class was to give a recital, I quit. I knew I was too fat to be dancing in front of an audience. When I was seven, my father—my hero, the understanding parent—died. Devastated by his death, food became my constant companion. It would surely never abandon me. Only food accepted me without question or demand.

My eating disorder and my weight grew over the years. I

had been introduced to diets before I was ten; in junior high, I was already a veteran dieter and used appetite suppressants.

I decided that by helping at home and excelling at school I could compensate for my personal deficiencies. Maybe if I worked hard enough, no one would notice how fat I was. I became responsible for styling my mother's hair, dressing myself and my sister, preparing meals, cleaning the house, shopping, and doing the laundry. Mom was the breadwinner, and it seemed only natural for me to become the little mother. Our lives settled into a routine.

I had few friends. More than once, my mother expressed concern about my isolation and lack of friends. "It's not normal for a child your age to spend all her time with adults. You should be with people your own age," she'd say. But I was more comfortable with adults. They didn't laugh at me or call me names. Adults always complimented me as the wonderful, helpful girl I was.

I developed health problems, though, and at thirteen had to have major surgery. I saw myself as even more defective after this, and I became completely isolated. My few outside activities were now unthinkable. Food was my only friend, and I was miserable.

Before the end of high school, I weighed 200 pounds. I looked and acted ten years older than I was. Suddenly, it seemed imperative that I lose weight. I developed the delusion that if I just lost weight and moved, life would improve. I secured college funding, went on a diet and, reached a normal weight for the first time. Things were now going to change. All my problems were solved!

While a freshman in college, I married and noticed that I could cope when the stress level was tolerable. When stress rose or there was any type of problem, I ate. I always placed blame for my difficulties and unhappiness outside myself, and I assumed the solution to also be external. My problems were because of my husband, my geographic location, my boss, God, the world. It was never my fault. I was the helpless victim.

Somehow, I finished college weighing only forty pounds more than when I began. My husband and I moved to a larger, more glamorous city, and I knew life had to get better. I was astonished that nothing seemed to change—except my weight. It continued to rise, and in two years I was back over 200 pounds. My pattern of disappointment, searching for a solution and blaming others continued.

Then, without warning, my husband left me. For the first time in my life, I couldn't eat. I was a real failure now. A period of agonizing indecision followed. Should I return to my family home where I had no job or stay where I was? I decided to stay. I divorced my husband, and over the next several months, lost weight. I had the solution now: My weight problems must have stemmed from my husband! With him out of the picture, I could certainly control my weight.

A friend soon introduced me to another man. After we had been dating a couple of months, he suggested we meet for a "discussion." I knew he was going to break off the relationship! Imagine my surprise when he explained that he disliked obesity in any form, but he liked me. I was fun, bright, interesting; however, would I please do something about the weight? I almost laughed. After all, I was down to only 165 from over two-hundred pounds. Of course I would do something about the weight! I already was! I continued to diet, reached my goal weight, and we became engaged.

Prior to our marriage, I solemnly promised him never to

gain weight again, but that proved impossible. We seemed happy, but even in the first year of marriage the eating compulsion started to get the best of me. One evening, I surreptitiously slipped the top of the wedding cake from the freezer, where we'd carefully stored it for our first anniversary, and consumed it over the kitchen sink. I meant to replace it, but waited too long! Oh, the humiliation when he found that empty box!

My weight began to mount. First ten, then twenty, then thirty pounds. I was despondent. Soon the whole world would know how inadequate I was. I'd start the day pulling my mask of calm competence into place, head for work, and return at night exhausted. I wondered why other people seemed to have so much energy, and I was always tired. I didn't realize the energy I wasted in maintaining this charade.

I tried everything: diet clubs, food plans, behavior modification, aversion therapy, exercise, health spas, and running. I became so compulsive about exercise and diet that my doctor accused me of being anorexic and said I must gain weight. All I could think was, "Boy, I wish I could get this on tape. No one will believe it!" But it didn't last.

A short time later I hit a rough spot in life. I couldn't seem to cope any longer. Although thin, I was bitterly unhappy. I began to eat, and in three years my weight doubled.

My husband didn't know what to do. At first he tried to support my attempts to lose weight, then gave up in frustration. My mood swings, depression, and anger were too much strain on our fragile relationship. When he suffered a back injury, I had to sleep in another room. After his back healed, he asked me to remain there. He didn't want close contact with me or my weight any longer.

I sought help and found none. I was unable to stick to a

diet for even one day. Weight loss became impossible. I spent every waking moment thinking about food: what to eat, when, how much. My weight soared to over two-hundred and forty pounds. How high it went, I'll never know; I just stopped weighing. I pretended not to understand why my clothes mysteriously shrank with every washing.

Despite my efforts to find help, the answer remained elusive. I became suicidal. In desperation, I decided to try one more counselor. This time fate, or God, took a hand. Instead of a careful search to find "the best," I simply picked a name at random out of the phone book and scheduled an appointment. Not ready for total honesty, I only admitted that my weight might be affecting my marriage. The second week, my counselor suggested Overeaters Anonymous. It took me three weeks to summon the courage to attend a meeting, but I knew that first night I was home.

Until then, I thought I was the only person who ate on the way home from work, then prepared and ate a full meal at home, or who ate at one fast food place, then another, and another. I thought I was the only one who hid deep sadness and loneliness beneath a facade of helpful cheerfulness.

I got a sponsor who helped me begin. We talked about the Steps, a Higher Power, and an inventory. I made a beginning and became abstinent. My inventory was written and given away. I attempted amends, tried to establish a relationship with God, and thought I was letting go of the defects. Relationships at home and work improved. I even had a few moments of happiness. It seemed this OA thing might work.

I lost about fifty pounds, but continued to experience enormous emotional pain. I had achieved a certain amount of relief, but was not yet in recovery. I had failed to let go of many character defects or to enlarge on my conscious contact with God. My selfish concerns eventually took over in the form of anger, self-pity, blame, resentment, and fear.

One of my major problems was that I was afraid of losing weight. This was so deeply buried that I didn't even know it. I had been sexually molested as a preteen, and my fat—along with clothes two sizes too big—was a camouflage I used to protect myself from men. When a male coworker attempted to compliment my emerging figure, he triggered this unrecognized fear, and I stopped losing weight.

At the next stressful point in life, I dove into relapse. I doubt it was a conscious choice, at first. But the second time I binged, I knew exactly what I was doing. I had not taken Step One, the full admission of my powerlessness. I fell for the illusion of being able to regain control whenever I chose.

In eighteen months of relapse, I regained all the weight I'd lost in the program and reached a new bottom. The only thing I did right during this time was attend meetings and give service. I believed recovery was possible in OA if I just "kept coming back." My sponsor, husband, and friends never gave up on me either. They continued to offer love and encouragement and on occasion reflected unpleasant truths to me.

Slowly, what I heard began to take hold. First was acceptance. I'd been angry with myself for my relapse. I finally began to accept that relapse was part of my process and to let go of the self-hatred. I accepted that God and others loved me. I was able to let them see the real me—not just the part I chose to show the rest of the world. With the understanding and support of my husband, sponsor, and friends, I slowly learned to love myself.

I accepted that, for me, recovery is learning to deal with all feelings: emotional and physical. While very young, I had

learned to suppress what I felt and became an expert at intel-
lectualizing. As I recovered, I started to experience feelings and
to let others know the pain and doubts I experienced. In time, I
was able to extend this to my physical body. I recognized that to
be fully alive, I had to exist in all three dimensions: spiritual,
emotional, and physical. That meant not only learning to
acknowledge my emotions, but also when I was tired, hungry,
thirsty, ill, or in pain.

A phrase that echoed frequently through my mind was,
"And we have ceased fighting anything and anyone—even
food." I quit trying to lose weight so quickly and found a food
plan I could live with, one day at a time, that allowed me to
achieve and maintain a healthy body size. I opted for a new way
of eating and of living.

When I quit fighting food, I became aware of the other
ways in which I fought recovery. I stopped blaming the rest of
the world, God, work, and my husband for "failing" me and
began to accept responsibility for my actions and my life.
Instead of running from God, I now wished to learn what God
wanted, and I attempted to follow God's will. To me, that meant
turning my thoughts and actions over to the care of God and
attempting to perform what I understood to be His will as best
I could. I'm not perfect, but I know that God understands and
forgives me. I try to do the same.

I finally stopped comparing myself to the rest of the world.
The other person always had more recovery or a better sponsor,
spiritual life, food plan, job, house, car, or husband.
Occasionally, I judged that I was in some way superior. I finally
learned that none of this matters. I learned humility. Being
myself was enough. I am neither better than nor less than anyone else. I can listen, learn, and keep an open mind, but com-

parisons had to stop!

Last, I learned about belief. I had always equated belief with faith. Through study, I discovered that belief means simply how we think. It comes before faith. When I act on belief, I think something will work. Faith happens after I have proven to myself that something is true. I heard someone say: "We become what we believe." Suddenly I realized I never thought I could recover. I became willing to believe in the possibility of success and recovery for myself.

Recovery didn't happen overnight. My emotional and spiritual growth coincided with my weight loss. For every pound lost, I grew in another area. Today, I'm not the same person who walked through the doors of OA over four years ago. I came into OA to lose weight and received so much more! None of the externals of my life changed. I still have the same husband, live in the same house, drive the same car, work at the same job. Yet everything inside me is different!

For the first time, I value and respect myself. I am loved, valued, and respected by others. I set limits and accept those set by others without taking them as personal rejection. I have a relationship with God and feel His presence in my life. I discovered that the God I thought deserted me years ago has been guiding and directing my life—even through all the years when I felt so alone and abandoned.

I have lost over one-hundred pounds and reached my goal weight. I look forward to many more years of continued growth and recovery. I can't simply maintain my recovery. I must move forward or lose what I have. I must practice the principles of the Twelve Steps every day, one day at a time. My adventure in life is just beginning!

16 _____

Negotiating Life's Curves

I AM ONE OF TWO sisters; my sister is six years older than I. My mother, my sister, and I are all compulsive eaters. I've been a compulsive overeater all my life.

I was a lonely child. I never felt that I fit in or that anyone liked me. I was always the last to be picked for team sports. My mother worked outside the home in an era when mothers stayed home and took care of their children; that too made me feel different.

From an early age I was more my mother's mother than she was mine. It was my responsibility to comfort her and make her feel all right. I sought the comfort and love I needed in food. When I felt bad (which was often), I ate. Although I felt fat as a child, I know today that I did not begin to gain weight until puberty. The feelings that were beginning to emerge terrified me, and I had no one to talk to. Food had always been there for me and was there then. I managed to get through school, feeling alone, different, and unliked. I passed all my classes and was even admitted to a state university, but I knew I was not very smart.

The summer after I graduated from high school, I found out about OA. My sister called me one day and announced that she had found the answer, and I must attend a meeting of Overeaters Anonymous. As she was my current and only Higher Power, I agreed to go. I didn't go because I wanted to stop eating. I went because I wanted to learn a way to eat whatever I wanted, whenever I wanted, and still be thin. Surely, there must be a way to do that.

At my first meeting, I didn't feel that I was home or that I had found an answer to my problem. What I did find was a diet (the "gray sheet") and a sponsor who had what I wanted: blonde hair, blue eyes, and a thin body. I began a pattern that would take me ten years to break: trying to abstain "perfectly" and failing, starting over and over again.

My first year, I had several sponsors and was not able to maintain perfect abstinence, but I did lose weight. Shortly after I completed my first year in program, I met the man who would become my husband. At the age of nineteen, I felt sure that no one else would ever love me and I better take him while I could.

Within three months of my marriage, I had gained thirty pounds and was pregnant. During that pregnancy my husband's drug use became overwhelming to both of us. We separated for a while and ultimately lost everything we had. My first son was born while we were living with my parents, the home I had so desperately wanted to be out of.

While I was pregnant, I lost thirty pounds. Within a few months, however, I was right back to where I was when I got pregnant. One year later, I got pregnant again. Again, I lost weight during my pregnancy, only to regain it all and more within a few months.

That marriage lasted five years. During that time, I attended meetings sporadically, as I was going to AA and it was much better than OA. After all, if you worked the steps in AA you could overcome any problem. I didn't need to go to OA, or so I thought. The problem with that thinking was I couldn't stop eating. I was powerless.

When my husband and I separated for the last time, I weighed 126 pounds after completing a diet and exercise program at a gym. Within three months, I had gained twenty-five pounds, and within six months I had gained fifty. I kept going to AA meetings and finding the people who felt like I did, that OA didn't work. We never discussed those of you who had stayed in OA and for whom this program was working. We stood around the food table at AA meetings and talked about how AA was a much better and stronger program. After all, it was the original Twelve-Step program. The problem was that I kept getting fatter, and worse than that, I hated myself. No matter what I tried, I couldn't stop eating.

That feeling of hopelessness (today I know that it was powerlessness) brought me back to OA. The leader at my first meeting back talked about the obsession as having a little man standing on my shoulder with a gun pointing at my head, saying, "If you don't eat, I will pull the trigger." For the first time I really understood what powerless meant.

That night I got down on my knees and asked God to remove the obsession. The obsession was removed (for a while), and I began to abstain. The first two years were difficult for me. A lot of the difficulty was that I was in denial about how difficult things were. I was a single mother of two small children, working full time, going to meetings, doing service, and pretending everything was all right. I returned to some of my old habits with food but not to bingeing the way I had. However, one night I made a conscious decision to break my abstinence and ate three cookies. Then I called a trusted friend in program and confessed. She asked me, "Aren't you tired of starting over?" I made another decision that night. I was never going to start over again; I date my continuous abstinence from that day, more than fifteen years ago.

After ten years in and out of OA, the beginning of abstinence was the letting go of perfection. I had to find success in each day and build on that, recognizing that each day was a gift from God, and my God didn't expect me to be more than human. Making a mistake did not mean I failed or that I was a failure. As I focused on my daily successes, they grew. Each day became a little easier than the last. So what has changed since then? Everything!

My food plan has changed too many times to remember since that day, but I have not returned to compulsive overeating. For that I am very grateful because it is truly the beginning of all other changes. Eliminating food allowed me to let God into my life in a way I never imagined possible. The "Big Book" promises that we will intuitively know how to handle situations that used to baffle us. My intuition, which got me into lots of trouble in the past, is today one of my best assets. Through trial and error, I have learned to trust my intuition, for that is most often how God speaks to me.

I learned that when faced with a decision or choice, I don't have to be afraid of making the wrong choice. There are no mistakes, just different lessons. I only have to listen to

God's voice to learn the lesson He has in store for me. I've learned that God's vision is far greater than mine. I began to see that life didn't revolve around me and that what happens to me doesn't take place in a vacuum. It is a great lesson that serves me still.

Writing dialogues with God is one of the greatest ways I have found to obtain and maintain conscious contact with my Higher Power. When writing a dialogue with God (it can also be written with anyone or anything you are experiencing difficulty with), God talks as much as or more than I do. I start out with my name and write whatever it is I have to say to or ask of God, and then I write "HP" or "God" and let my Higher Power speak. My first thought about this form of writing was, "Come on, it is my hand and my pen doing the writing; it will just be my will that ends up on the paper." But I was willing, tried it, and found that there were two voices on that piece of paper, God's and mine.

By practicing this type of communication with God, I found that I developed a much stronger sense of God's presence in my life. I was better able to "hear God's voice" through my instincts, the way in which God most often speaks to me. I also found that it is important to read this writing to someone else.

My relationships have changed dramatically since I began to abstain. My sons were five and seven when I began my abstinence. My relationship with them consisted of yelling and hitting. They were afraid of me, and the love I expressed to them was confusing. At a retreat, one of my OA friends told me that I had "screwed up" and asked me what I was going to do about it. It was the first time someone told me that I had to take responsibility for my actions. Previously, everyone had told me that I was doing the best I could. As long as I believed that, I felt guilty but didn't feel I had to change. Being responsible for my actions eliminated the guilt and allowed me to begin changing my behavior.

The changes in our relationship were gradual and slow. Like my own growth, I continue to see improvement. Those little boys are now men. My older son has been on his own for several years. He has been sober for more than a year and changing every day. We talk on the phone frequently as he lets me know what is going on in his life. He trusts me and today can feel the great love I have for him. My younger son still lives at home. He has been sober for more than two years. I was privileged to take him to his first AA meeting.

My current husband and I met early in the year I began to abstain. We have had many struggles over the years, but we continue to grow together and learn to trust each other. He is not in the program, and I once felt that he didn't understand. Today, I know that is not true. In the early days of our relationship, I was insecure and felt that the only way I could have love was to find it and hold on for dear life. I didn't have a sense of independence. We lived together and married, but we didn't know how to talk to each other, and there was not much trust. We have been in therapy together over the years. We learned to communicate and to see that we didn't have to be alike to like each other. We learned that we could each bring our strengths into the relationship and learn from each other. We didn't need to always enjoy doing the same things, but we could share the joy of the other's activities.

More recently, we learned to really talk and listen to each other. I have learned that I am safe with him and can be vulnerable. I can tell him anything and know that he will listen and try to understand. He not only listens to my words, but also to my feelings.

Three years ago the message was very clear from my Higher Power that it was time for my family and me to move away from the only city I remember living in. The prospect was a scary one, but I felt directed. The gut feeling that told me it was time, and following that feeling all the way through, proved to me once again that God does indeed work in my life.

Today, I am in the process of changing jobs. The first two jobs after our move were disastrous. They paid the bills but at a very high price. When the doctor told me that the stress was more than my body could handle and that I had better leave my job, I realized that God was telling me it was time for another change. I began career counseling and investigating career possibilities.

When I came into OA at age eighteen, I believed that I was not very smart. After my divorce from my first husband, God led me to a job that turned into a career. Finding something I liked and was good at gave me the self-esteem I never had before. Over the years, I have come to see that I am indeed smart. I believe that God will direct me to a job where I can be of the most use to God and to my fellows.

I feel that all I've learned, I've learned in this program. I have learned by living each day. I learn every time I make a mistake. I learn every time I fall down and pick myself up. I learn every time I take two steps forward and one step back. Of course, I learn from my everyday life and all the experiences I have. However, I wonder if I would be open to life's lessons without the knowledge and faith I have acquired by living this program. It has given me all the tools I need.

Today, I envision my journey as going up a mountain.

Sometimes I can't see ahead because of the curves. I can look back and see how far I've come and know that the road ahead will be safe if I continue to travel with my Higher Power and my friends. As I go up the mountain, I look down at the valley below. Each time I come around a curve I have a different perspective, as I am a little higher up than I was last time around. What that means to me is that I continue to learn the same lessons, but each time with a different view and at a deeper level. As long as I don't have to travel alone, I won't be afraid of the heights I will reach, and I won't take credit for reaching them alone.

17

Opening the Doors and Closets

FOOD WAS ALWAYS IMPORTANT in our family. Food was the means by which love could be shown without ever saying the word out loud. My mother or grandmother could show their love by baking a large cobbler, and I could return that love by eating a lot of it. I learned early on about the power of food. Later I was to learn its real power and how to use it to kill the pain in my life. It was to become my drug of choice. I was the loner, scared of people, but really wanting them in my life more than anything. Food helped me deal with that fear of people, but later it turned on me and led me into even deeper fear, isolation, and loneliness.

I don't believe that I really crossed over the line between normal eating and compulsive overeating until I was fourteen. It was then that I began to use food to survive the pain and fear that took over my life. One of the relatives responsible for my emotional and sexual abuse died suddenly. I also had a major operation and feared I would die. I became aware that I was different from the other boys. I knew even then that I was gay, even though I did not have a word for it.

All these things coming together crossed me over that thin line between normal eating and compulsive overeating. I went from weighing sixty to eighty pounds at fourteen to weighing around 300 pounds at age seventeen. Unconsciously, I used my addiction to survive and not kill myself until God knew I could face that pain and fear with His help.

Over the years, no matter what my weight, I was never okay inside. In 1983, at age thirty-nine, I wanted to die because I was in so much emotional pain. My successful business of six years was going down the drain because of my craziness. I was screaming and throwing things at employees. And my food was out of control. However, I still held to the ideal that everything would be okay if I were thin. This in spite of the fact that even when I was thin before, I was still lonely and afraid inside.

In May of 1983, I was entering people's lives like a hurricane and leaving like a tornado, leaving them a wreck—bleeding and crying. I wanted to hurt people because of my own pain, fear, and anger. In the early moments after I awakened, still somewhere between sleeping and being fully awake, I would either say the Lord's Prayer or think about shooting myself with the gun in the drawer next to the bed. Two strange people who didn't drink no matter what (recovering alcoholics) saw through my many masks and started to Twelfth-Step me in OA by telling me those magic words: "Friends of ours in OA lost a lot of weight." I was too scared to go, however, because I didn't think it would work for me, and I feared people terribly. I had to wait until God knew I was ready. Even then, it took a lot to get my attention and make me willing to break through the fear and pain, no matter what.

One Saturday in May 1983, I was at my lowest point emotionally and spiritually. Driving on a freeway, drinking a soda, and eating candy, I came upon a parked car in my lane and hit it at forty to fifty miles an hour, not wearing a seat belt. It took several years before I honestly realized that I could have avoided the collision by simply changing lanes. Today I know that at that moment, I decided to kill myself and end the pain. I walked away without a bruise, however. On Monday, my doctor told me I wasn't hurt because I was so fat, but he said I needed to lose weight for health reasons. I told him that I had been thinking about going to Overeaters Anonymous. At that instant, I took the first step without knowing it existed. I was totally powerless and my life was utterly unmanageable. I went home and told my friends that I wanted to go to a meeting on Friday night.

On Friday, May 27, 1983, I walked into my first meeting. Before the hour was over, I knew that I was where I belonged. Most of my life had been spent alone and full of overwhelming and paralyzing fear, anger, guilt, and shame. I never believed I could find a solution until I walked into these rooms.

In these rooms, I heard people laughing about the way I felt inside, but they were laughing because they no longer felt that way. I wanted that. I wanted the laughter and hugs because I had had neither in my life for years. I had just sat at home with the blinds pulled, watched TV, and ate more and more. I couldn't stop eating once I started. I was still scared, but I was in so much pain that I was willing to try anything. I heard that you eat three meals a day, nothing in between, and no sugar. And that you were only as sick as your secrets.

I read some of the literature that night and decided to try to eat only three meals and no sugar the next day. The next day I went to a family reunion. I made the mistake of telling them I was on a diet, so all weekend they talked about what I could or couldn't eat. The miracle is that I ate three meals, nothing in between, and no sugar. For me this was my Second Step, since I knew that only God could have done that for me. I have been abstinent since that day.

Speaking of God, that concept alone almost made me leave before I started. Early in my childhood, I had a loving, caring God. I even wanted to be a minister. But somewhere about the time I crossed over into compulsive eating, my God changed. He became a vengeful, unloving God who could not accept me as I was. I asked the two people who brought me to that first meeting if OA was a cult or a religion, because there seemed to be a lot of chanting and praying at the meeting. I was afraid that their God would not accept me and give me what I saw in the people there. They told me not to worry, to just keep coming back and the God thing would work itself out. At first, I had to fake having a God, and I made the group my Higher Power. Later I found a path through the Steps back to the loving and caring God that I had as a nine year old. He is my God today, and I thank Him before every meal and on my knees every night for giving me abstinence and loving relationships in my life.

After three to four months of abstinence, losing weight, and going to a lot of meetings, I came to a major crisis—my secrets. I knew I had to tell my deepest, darkest, most ugly secret to the two people who had brought me into the program or eat compulsively again. So one day I decided to tell them my secret over lunch (seems I used to do everything over or after food). I couldn't do it. Then after lunch in the car, God gave me the courage to tell them, my first straight friends ever, that I was gay. They simply said, "We know; we still love you." That was for me a spiritual experience of the burning bush type. By deciding to tell them, I truly trusted God for the first time and became willing to turn my life over to Him and trust He would take care of me no matter what. I had taken the Third Step. I then knew that I would always be okay as long as I continued to trust Him. That was the first step to being able to deal with my sexuality and to begin the road to being comfortable with myself. It has been the longest and most difficult journey of my life and one that is not yet complete. Today I am openly gay and free to be me with everyone in my life including my family, friends, and business associates.

That freedom let me feel the pain of working the Steps and helped me incorporate them into my daily life. The Steps were painful for me because for the first time I had to face the pain I always avoided. The Steps have helped me live through the pain without eating it away. It has helped me to understand that no matter what, good or bad, "this too shall pass."

Over the past seventeen years, I have never had a perfect abstinence, but I have never eaten like I used to eat or gone back to the sugar. Perfection for me is a killer. I can never be perfect; only God is perfect. I have had enough shame in my life that I don't need to shame myself over not having a perfect abstinence. As long as I am abstinent today, my goal weight is what I weigh today. I don't worry about it because I can't change my weight one day at a time. Only God can do that instantly, and if I'm abstinent, my weight is exactly what God wants it to be today. Weight is not the problem. Life is the problem, and I work on that through the Twelve Steps and daily contact with my God.

If I am abstinent, I can look and listen to see whom God has put in my life to tell me His will for me. As the "Big Book" says, "nothing happens in God's world by accident," so the people in my life are not there by accident. They are there to tell me something, so I need to stop my addictions long enough to hear them.

Early in my abstinence, angry over a small incident, I stopped at a store to buy a diet soda. Instead, however, I began to think about not if I would eat an ice cream bar, but how many I would eat. Sitting in my car, a moment of clarity, as the "Big Book" describes it, came to me when a woman who was apparently a compulsive overeater came out of the store. She stopped in front of my car at a trash can and pulled an ice cream bar from her bag. She wolfed it down and pulled another from the bag and did the same. In that moment of clarity, I knew that God had just told me that I did not have to compulsively overeat that day. Today I know that by opening my eyes and ears to the people around me, I find God's message of recovery if I stop for a minute before I take that first compulsive bite.

God in His time has given me the people to help me deal with my sexuality, incest, sexual abuse, AIDS issues, low self-esteem, and depression. As the issues have come up, people have been there to help me. If I work the program, I believe that no matter how depressed I feel or how much pain I'm in, God gives me the tools and the people with which to go through it without eating. I am not unique; others in this program have shown me that.

A lot of what I say and do today, I first heard about in the rooms of OA. I find that amazing because when I first came to

OA, I thought that no one else had the secrets or problems I had. This uniqueness, like perfection, almost killed me. I thought that my only problem was that I was fat and I couldn't stop eating. If at that point I had limited myself to only being thin, I would have cheated myself out of most of the benefits of the program. Today I only feel unique when I am in the "dis-ease" of the disease and want to stay in my own self-pity. This feeling of self-pity and uniqueness will, if unchecked, lead me to once again believe there is no solution except food. That is why I must continue to work the Steps and form a support group that will honestly and lovingly confront me when I begin to get back into the disease.

Among the winners in this program are not only those who maintain long-term abstinence, but also those who keep coming back no matter what. As long as I keep coming back, I have a chance. I don't care what road of recovery you take. There are many paths to the same recovery. I am not God, so I can't choose yours. You may work the Steps to get abstinent or get abstinent to work the Steps. The important thing for me is that you keep coming back to give me the knowledge that it can be done, and I can do the same should I ever binge again or leave the program. I must remember that for me the only important thing is to keep coming back no matter what.

Diets never worked for me. I always used drugs to lose weight before I came to OA. My last major weight loss before OA was in 1978. For eight to nine months, I had only a bowl of vegetable soup, a glass of iced tea, and a lot of valium dropped into three or four scotches a day. I was thin, but crazy, and the black void inside of me from childhood still festered. When being thin stopped working, I started to eat once again. Today that void is slowly being filled spiritually.

Today I have to be who I am openly and freely and accept that I am exactly who God wants me to be as long as I try to do His will daily. I reached the point where the pain of eating was greater than the emotional pain I was trying to kill, and I gave up the compulsive eating. God took care of me by giving me a program to deal with that pain. After many years, I still use the same tools. I go to meetings, read literature, associate with recovering people, work the Steps, and get down on my knees and ask God every night to keep me abstinent. No matter what, I don't compulsively overeat, one day at a time. For me, the program has made my life better, then worse, then better, then worse, then better. . . . As the most hateful line in the "Big Book" says, "More shall be revealed." Through the Steps and the program, I have learned to deal with the new pain and go on with my life. It has ups and downs and pain and joy. For me, food will never solve problems or eliminate pain. OA has not been the end of the road of recovery for me, but the beginning. The Steps and the program have taught me to live again and take the risks to do anything necessary to stay on the road, including such things as therapy and other programs to deal with the problems I used to eat over. All OA promised me was that I didn't have to eat compulsively or be alone again. It has, however, done even more by opening the doors and closets of my mind to allow me to deal with every aspect of my life and to find freedom from pain and fear.

Before I came into the program, I tried to fill a spiritual void with the physical act of eating. Today, OA has given me a loving and caring God to fill that void. I know now that my God will always take care of me if I just let Him.

18 _____

I Made Out My
Will at Twenty-Two

I WAS A FAT KID, and I went through all
the horrors of growing up as a fat kid in a fat-phobic society,
from wearing "husky" sizes, to being called names, to being
picked last for sports teams. I went on my first diet when I was
ten years old, motivated mainly by the dollar a pound that my
mother promised me for losing weight. I managed to lose
about thirty pounds, which was about half of what I needed to
lose. However, one day I got sidetracked by a "special occasion" and couldn't seem to get back on my diet; it seemed like
every day turned into a special occasion. I don't have any
excuses for why I ate—my parents did not beat me, and I was
spared the "children are starving in Africa" stories that many
other children heard.

I tried a variety of self-imposed remedies over the years,
from diets to exercise plans to cross-country moves. I learned
the hard way that the geographic cure did not work for me. I

just brought my problems with me wherever I went. I, who hated physical education classes, went out for football thinking that the forced exercise would fix me. I ended up with a torn ligament. I thought that becoming an all-natural, long-haired Grateful Deadhead would fix me. It didn't. I thought that cutting my hair off and getting a "real job" would fix me. It didn't. I always seemed to think that the diet I started next Monday morning would fix me, but I found myself bingeing by mid-afternoon. I even went through a stage of being a "liberated" fat person. After reading those stories that say most diets fail and most fat children become fat adults, I decided to give up on losing weight. I figured that as long as I was doomed to be fat, I might as well eat whatever I wanted. Sure, I thought, I might gain a few pounds, but at least my body would find its natural set point. I figured that I would find that set point, accept myself at that weight, and live happily ever after.

Sixty-five pounds later I realized that my set point was set at infinity, since I kept gaining weight and couldn't stop. I had passed from the realm of just being fat into the realm of being morbidly obese. I couldn't find clothing in normal clothing stores, and my health was deteriorating. Personal hygiene became difficult because it was hard to reach certain places to clean. Climbing a flight of steps became a major physical exertion. Stretch marks advanced down my arms and across my belly. My blood pressure was climbing to the warning level, and then came the chest pains. I remember the nights I was having chest pains and thought I was having a heart attack. I wondered if I would live through the night. So I did what any normal twenty-two-year-old would do in my situation: I was too embarrassed to call a doctor, so I made out my will. The doctor might find out I was fat.

By the way, I was a closet overeater. Although I am sure that everyone could tell what I was doing with food by looking at my forty-six-inch waist, I did my most industrial strength bingeing in private. I thought that if other people didn't see me eat, it didn't count. I would shop at different grocery stores on different days so the clerks would not see how much junk food I was eating. I would buy vegetables to go along with the candy, since that would make the trip to the market "legitimate" and disguise (so I thought) the amount of food I was really eating. Of course, the vegetables would die of old age in the refrigerator.

My insanity was such that I would binge on the way home from the big man's shop. I knew that my overeating was killing me, but I could not stop. Sometimes when I was bingeing the food didn't even taste good, and it hurt to eat more. Still I could not stop. I would tell myself that I would have just one more bite and stop, but I never stopped until all the food was gone.

Out of desperation, I crawled into Overeaters Anonymous. Right away I got a sponsor who suggested that I go to ninety Overeaters Anonymous meetings in ninety days. She also suggested that I stop eating my binge foods, eat three meals a day, and call her every morning to tell her what I planned to eat that day. I was very confused by OA meetings at first, since I was so fogged out on food that I could not understand a lot of the jargon that I heard. However, I could see that OA worked for many people, and I figured that if I did what worked for them, then it would work for me. Since I did not understand the words, I focused on the actions that other people had taken to get better. I listened to their stories, talked to them after meetings, and called them on the telephone. I wanted to know what actions they had taken, what meetings they attended, what service jobs they held, and what they ate. At first I expected that the ones who were getting better in the program had some kind of strange secret, like a magic vitamin supplement; but then one day at a meeting I noticed that all the people who were getting well had one thing in common: they were working the Twelve Steps of Overeaters Anonymous. That included not just the ten of the twelve that are identical to the corresponding AA Steps, but the two that are very different in Overeaters Anonymous. In Step One we admit that we are powerless over food, and in Step Twelve we carry the message to other compulsive overeaters. They were also using all eight tools of recovery that we use as part of working the Steps. I also noticed that those who were still struggling were usually not working one or more of the Steps or tools.

I did not make ninety OA meetings in those next ninety days. I probably only made about eighty. However, it was good enough, and I learned one of OA's great lessons: that good enough is good enough. I don't have to be perfect anymore. Perfectionism is a trap left over from my dieting days, when I had to be either perfectly starving myself or perfectly bingeing.

OA took 110 pounds off my body in the next year, and by the grace of this program I have been maintaining that weight reduction for more than nine years. It is a joy to discard clothes because they wear out, not because I have outgrown them. Reaching a normal size for the first time in my life was a major readjustment. I had thought all my problems would be solved if only I lost weight. I thought when I hit my goal weight I would be a six-foot-tall millionaire with a body that looked like an Olympic swimmer's. I discovered that when I reached my goal weight, I was still short, still had to work for a living, and still had lots of loose skin and stretch marks. The stretch marks have faded a bit after nine years, but they are still there, and my skin is still loose in places.

Even though I have been abstaining for over ten years, I am still a compulsive overeater. I am not cured. I need to continue working the OA program. In the morning, I get on my knees and ask God for help. Then I take a few moments and try to meditate. I call my sponsor almost every day and hear from my sponsorees regularly. I go to a lot of OA meetings because I have discovered that when I get to a lot of meetings, it is easy for me to eat properly. When I don't get to a lot of OA meetings—even if I am getting to one of the many other Twelve-Step programs that I qualify for—it is harder for me to eat properly. I have a service job at an OA meeting because it gets me there and because I have noticed that people who do committed service jobs at meetings have an easier time of it than people who don't. I eat three meals a day with nothing in between, because that seems to work for me. I don't eat the foods that cause problems for me, and that includes not only candy and sweets but also a few starchy foods such as bread, rice, and potatoes. I discovered over several years of experimentation in OA that these foods just did not work for me, although they may work for other compulsive overeaters. I also have to pay attention to portion control, since my natural appetite is about as accurate as my natural vision—about 20/800. Just as I need glasses to help me see well, I need the tools and Steps of the OA program to help me eat properly.

By the way, I have since updated my will to add my lovely wife, whom I met in OA, the child we are expecting, and a modest bequest to Overeaters Anonymous. I came to OA so I wouldn't die from obesity. I never expected to find such a wonderful way of life. Keep coming back. It keeps on working.

19

It Wasn't Fair

IT JUST WASN'T FAIR. I was sixteen years old and weighed almost 300 pounds. I don't really know how I got there. It was as if I were living in a nightmare for sixteen years and suddenly woke up, fat and afraid. I cried all the time, but could never really explain why. I was tired of diets and sick of trying to lose weight.

My life was given over to food: hiding it, sneaking it, then counting calories and trying every new fad diet that came along. My sole purpose in life seemed to be to lose weight. I would vow to become a certain weight or a certain size before the next school year or the next birthday, only to fail again. That was my life. I was miserable. I still shudder to remember what it was like in those days.

I remember how awful it felt to be the youngest and fattest wherever I went. In public and at family gatherings, I was acutely conscious of my size and my age. I was always the one with the charming personality.

"If only she would lose weight, she would be adorable," the aunts and other relations would cluck. They never intended to hurt my feelings. But I was very good at hiding my feelings.

Actually, my best friends and strongest supporters were my family and their friends. It seems strange, but the people closest to me were all much older than I. Now I know that it was because I was ridiculed and re rejected by my peers. Kids can be so cruel.

I still remember the all-school assembly in sixth grade when I was initiated into safety patrols. Every one laughed when that fluorescent orange belt wouldn't fit around me. Or the time in the junior high school cafeteria when my classmates threw peanuts at me, and choruses of "Dumbo!" echoed through the lunchroom.

But the most painful time of all was in the tenth grade when the class yearbook came out. There was a full-page picture of me, close to 300 pounds, leaning against a tree. The caption identified me by name, and joked in print that I was "holding up the tree."

But kids aren't the only ones who lack compassion. It took me a long time to ride a bike again after the man who lived around the corner called me over just to say hello, then proceeded to laugh hysterically about the way the bike tires would flatten to the rim every time I sat down.

The utter humiliation of that fat! The first time I ever undressed in the locker room, the other girls laughed and joked and pointed to the rolls and layers of blubber. They thought they were teasing; I'm sure they didn't intend to be so cruel. But I never gave them another chance to hurt me like that. From that day on, I always wore my gym shorts and T-shirt under my clothes. My school clothes were a uniform, anyway: stretch pants and a knit top. What did it matter if I added another layer? Not many stylish clothes for teenagers come in size forty-six and forty-eight. There were no gym suits large enough to fit me, of course, and I never could wear a Girl Scout uniform. I was the only girl in my troop without one. I also was the only student in my high school hospital careers class without the traditional white coat. They didn't have one large enough. Teachers didn't help, either. It was humiliating enough to have to dress differently from the other kids for gym class, but then the teacher would send me off by myself in an auxiliary gym with nothing to keep me company but a boring "inches off" exercise book. They wouldn't let me participate in games or sports. I guess they thought I might keel over.

Thank God for the few good friends I had during this period. The ones who liked me then, in spite of what I looked like, are the ones I know will always be dear to me.

Although it was food that was making my life so miserable all those years, it always appeared to be my friend. Or so I thought. It kept me company, relieved anxiety and covered up everything I ever felt. Food interfered with living. I can see now I wasn't living, merely existing—and miserably.

It is strange to realize when I look back that I was trying to "get even" with my friends, and especially my family, by eating. How it hurt them to see me eating and apparently not caring what I was doing to myself. I overlooked the fact that although I was hurting them, I was destroying myself.

I hated what I was doing. The games I played for so long were becoming meaningless. I was tired of cleverly devising new ways to cover up what I ate. I had become an expert at eating as much ice cream as possible without letting the bottom of the carton show through. I thought I fooled everyone by not chewing whatever was in my mouth if someone walked into the room unexpectedly.

The only good thing I remember about being fat—at least I considered it positive at the time—was that being obese gave me an unreal sense of power. I was bigger, and my fat made me feel more powerful than my peers. I didn't feel like a girl at all. I had to lose more than a hundred pounds before I felt any sense of femininity. In my fat days I didn't care about my appearance. All I ever wore were big shirts and pants that would stretch, and boys' tennis shoes. I never washed or combed my hair. It's hard to believe I once lived like such a slob, but it's true. My mother tried to help me. She took me to a popular diet club four different times, the first time when I was only ten years old. I did fairly well on their diet, but I always stopped going after the fifteenth week. I couldn't face that award ceremony which came on the sixteenth week, when you had to walk up in front of a large group of people to receive a pin. I could never bring myself to do that.

When I was thirteen or fourteen, a friend introduced me to another weight-loss group. I was successful there for short periods of time, but I don't remember feeling as if they really cared about me. That was true in the first diet club too.

I guess it was about this same time that the school nurse suggested I visit the public school psychologist. My parents, who all along would have given anything for me to lose weight, agreed I should go. For the next two years I met with a doctor every Wednesday after noon. I suppose he tried, but he never really understood how I felt. Each counseling session became a contest to see if I could cry louder than he yelled.

"It's not that difficult," he would scream at me. "You just don't give a damn!" If he only could have known how very much I cared.

I cared enough to try acupuncture next, a drastic step. I was positive this was the answer. I didn't know a whole lot about it, but at that point I was near the end of my rope and so was my family. After a long family discussion about the cost of acupuncture treatment—and some caustic comments about my determination to stick with it—we decided to give it a whirl. It cost more than $100 to have the staple inserted in my ear, and ten dollars a week for the treatment. But it wasn't long before I simply stopped going. Interestingly enough, the acupuncture treatment worked well physically. It did decrease my appetite. But it did not decrease my intake of food. I ate whether I was hungry or not.

To this day I don't really know why I came to OA. I was sure I was destined to be fat forever. I read about OA in the newspaper, and one Thursday night I made my way to a meeting. I don't know what made me go. I do know I didn't like it. I have no memory of the speaker, topic, or discussion. All I saw at that meeting was the tops of my shoes. I never looked up, but tried to hide my tears by hanging my head. I still remember the way the teardrops beaded on the tops of my shoes, never really sinking in. The OA philosophy didn't sink in, either—at least not that night.

It took only about a half hour of that torture for me to decide that OA wasn't for me. I ran from the room, leaving the meeting in the middle of the discussion, wiping my teary eyes and hoping against hope that my mother and sister would come by early to pick me up.

I stood there in the dark by the curb, utterly alone, depressed and feeling that once again a group had failed me. No one cared.

But that's where OA people are different from any I had ever known before. I heard footsteps behind me. I didn't know who it was, but I knew she was from the OA group inside. She didn't know me, had no personal reason for following me outside. She just came to give me a hug, assure me she cared, and hoped I would come back. If she had not made that effort to reach out to me, to take the time to tell me more about the program, I know I would have added OA to my list of failures. I'll always remember what she did for me that night, and I'll always be grateful.

Through that caring person, I found a sponsor, a beautiful person. She not only was—and is—a super sponsor, but our relationship has grown and blossomed into a caring and trusting friendship.

Nobody else would have put up with what I put her through. She never complained. She spent many hours patiently explaining how the program works. My first few weeks in OA were spent on an erratic on-again, off-again abstinence. But that was OK. My sponsor was patient, loving and understanding. I could sense her caring, her willingness to share what I needed. One Thursday night I was talking with her on the phone as usual, only this conversation was different. I broke down, crying my heart out, pouring out my feelings of worthlessness and confusion.

"Stop!" she said suddenly. "We've got to talk. I want you to meet me in front of the church where your OA meeting is."

It was a bitter cold, icy night, and she drove all the way down from the opposite end of the county. I couldn't understand why anyone would come so far on such a night for me, but I went and met her. That was the first time I had met her in person, and that was my first day of abstinence. I have been abstinent ever since, more than a year now. It was through her support, and the help and guidance of many others like her that I have been able to maintain a good, strong, unshakable abstinence—and a weight loss of more than 111 pounds so far.

During my first six months in the program, I felt as if I were being tested over and over again. I refused to go to parties in the beginning because I was afraid I'd lose my abstinence. I couldn't handle the food choices. Eventually, I didn't hurt so much and could handle holidays and family gatherings without overeating, or even being tempted to overeat.

Some of these family occasions seemed interminable. I remember my uncle's birthday party, where I spent half the evening locked in the bathroom with a box of Kleenex and the telephone I had pulled through the door.

How clearly my sponsor spoke to me that night, reminding me of my own responsibility, and assuring me that I was capable of making the right choices. Again that night, she comforted me with those simple words I've heard so often and still need to hear: "It's going to be all right. Just continue to follow the program."

My sponsor never failed me on those occasions when I needed to talk, to be reassured. I called her from parties, from restaurants, from school, from wherever I was, for whatever I needed. A few weeks after that night came my birthday. I know birthdays are supposed to be happy occasions, but I was new in the program. And I was only seventeen years old. I felt deprived without that traditional birthday cake with candles. It just wasn't fair that I had to give up an old birthday tradition for a new way of life that was not yet comfortable.

How my feelings and my lifestyle changed over the next few months!

One night I was having dinner out with friends when I had one of those insights that come from the OA program. I suddenly realized—for the first time—that I simply couldn't eat the same way as most of my friends. But I didn't resent it or in any way feel deprived. It was just a fact of life.

I excused myself and quickly ran to a public telephone phone to call my sponsor. She had helped me through so much, patiently talked me through so many bad times, that it was only fair that I also share my growth and joy with her, too.

That night was exciting. I went to sleep feeling on top of the world. So what if I couldn't eat certain foods! I was just beginning to wake up and live in a world that before OA was only a fantasy. Food no longer ruled my life. I was free. I had recently bought my very first pair of pants with pockets and a zipper (instead of an elastic waistband). I had passed my driver's test and had my operator's license. My family and friends were thrilled about my weight loss. People cared about me, and I cared for them. And I honestly cared about myself. I came to understand that if I eat compulsively I'm not being fair to myself.

Then I finally realized that it wasn't life all those years that hadn't been fair to me; it was I who hadn't been fair to myself. That was something I could change, and right then I decided I would.

I did change and grow in lots of ways from that point on. Some changes and growth came unexpectedly and tragically. When I had been in the program less than a year, my mother died suddenly. One day she was there, and the next she wasn't.

The pain was acute, and the wound deep. It took a long time to heal, but food wasn't part of the medication. My Higher Power and my OA friends gave me the strength to work through the grief and survive, a stronger person. I know now that my finding OA when I did was no coincidence, and that my very special sponsor was a gift—the right person in the right place at the right time.

The night before my mother died, she and I had gone to an OA meeting together. I was so proud of her, and I know she was proud of me. I feel great comfort in knowing she died abstinent. I truly believe it was God's way of showing me the importance of OA in my life.

I know that as long as I follow the OA program, everything I must face in life will turn out all right, and my life will be as fair to me as I allow it to be.

20

Sink the Lollipop!

IN A FAMILY OF TEN children, I was number nine and the only girl. My father left us when I was a year old, and my brothers, never short of playmates, did not deign to play with a girl. At the age of eleven, I was sexually molested.

It does not seem far-fetched to suspect that these experiences made me wary of the male sex. Now in my fifties, I feel I have not been able to trust men enough to want one for a husband. Boyfriends I have had; a permanent relationship, never.

It was well before I entered my teens that I began to build my ship. I made it out of pure chocolate, and it was my sanctuary for thirty-nine years. Aboard my ship, I worked my way up to ten to twenty candy bars a day plus a variety of other chocolate concoctions. By the age of sixteen I had reached 240 pounds.

Within the huge body was an emotionally contorted child. When things got out of hand, as they usually did, I expected people to look after me. I grew angry with God when He would not do as I wished and turned to the medical profession, demanding that doctors do for me what God wouldn't.

I set impossible goals for myself and became angry when I didn't reach them. But candy solved all my problems. It relieved depressions, eliminated the need to make decisions and was a handy, all-purpose reward, as appropriate for failure as for success.

Many times I ventured out of my magic ship, vowing never to return. But I always did. I was safe there and no one else could come aboard to criticize me. During my brief absences I visited many doctors. They all said the same thing, "Lose weight or else." I did; in fact, I went up and down as regularly as the waves in the ocean. It began to be clear to me that death was not going to wait until I grew old to claim me. But I really didn't care. I had decided by this time that I would die on my ship and die happy. I did not realize how long it takes or how painful it would be.

When I contracted rheumatoid arthritis at the age of thirty, the doctor asked me, "Have you gone through an emotional crisis recently?"

"My whole life has been an emotional crisis," I replied.

My condition of psychic chaos was on slow simmer until one June day when I was told that I would die if I didn't lose weight. (As if I didn't know.) I was also informed that there was now a way to lose weight which didn't require will power. It was a surgical procedure called the intestinal bypass. Out of everything the doctor said, I heard only " You can eat and still lose weight" and "You will have a lot of diarrhea."

I waited until my weight reached 308 pounds and then submitted to the operation. Thus began eight years of hell. The lowest point my weight reached after the bypass was 240 pounds. Then it began to yo-yo. I had diarrhea so badly I could not leave the house for a whole year. I finally got so I could control this condition somewhat, and then the flatulence started. It was very degrading.

After three years, I started having kidney trouble. I underwent two operations for the removal of stones and then a third to remove a kidney. That was the beginning of a five-year ordeal during which I had twenty-five operations, eleven related to the damaged kidney.

I suffered acute attacks of pain which the doctors could not explain. I had rashes and allergies. I was extremely short-winded and could hardly move about. The only social life I had was visiting doctors and, occasionally, my family.

Three days after my kidney was removed the doctors told me I had to have the bypass reversed or I would develop trouble with the other kidney, in which case I would have less than three years to live. I decided at this point that it was too painful to die. Still, I could not give up my only solace. I retreated to my ship. I ate because I was sick, and I was sick because I ate.

Eight years after the bypass was performed, it was reversed with the warning that I had no chance of pulling through. But again I was saved, though it seemed to me that death would have been better. I felt only pain. Nothing else. Now I was convinced that I had lost my last chance of ever being thin. I had tried everything and there was absolutely nowhere else to go.

As if on cue, the incision opened up and became infected. It drained for four months. The doctors gave up and said it would drain the rest of my life.

It was imperative now to blot out my situation. My weight climbed back up to 291 pounds. Suddenly, I became aware of what I was doing. I knew I did not want to reach the 300-pound mark again. For the first time I said, "God, help me! "

On Valentine's Day I received what I had asked for in the form of a telephone number a friend had given me more than two years earlier. I had put it in a drawer and forgotten it. I called the number and on the day of love I hobbled into my first OA meeting. I could hardly walk across the room. I was told later that they didn't know if they were going to have to carry me out after the meeting. I was a mess physically and emotionally.

But at that very first meeting I saw a ray of hope. I went to another meeting the next night and I started abstaining the following day. On that day, the incision which the doctors said would drain the rest of my life stopped draining and began to heal.

Out of the total desperation in which I came, I was willing to accept anything OA had to offer. I did not understand much of what was going on, but I knew I wanted what I saw. I started the program by doing everything I was supposed to do: abstaining, speaking, volunteering for service, writing and giving away my inventory, becoming a sponsor. I went to as many meetings as possible and worked the Steps to the best of my ability. It took me four months to begin to understand what I was doing.

I had felt for years that I had lost my faith. I could not ask God for anything because He never heard me. Then one night I was told, "Action is the magic word," and I found that I had not lost my faith. It had been there all the time, waiting for me to start acting on it. Once I started the action, things got better. Now I am learning to take responsibility for myself. I have found a small part of me. I know I am a human being and a child of God. That is a wonderful thing to know. It's so much better than being a "freak of nature." I am aware that my life was an emotional crisis because I let it be.

My physical problems are beginning to disappear. I grow stronger every day. I now sail into meetings (I leave my cane at home). At one meeting I climb two flights of stairs. I read all the literature I can get my hands on and enjoy every word. I let my Higher Power run my life and, friends, you cannot believe the things I accomplish in twenty-four hours. I visit people in the hospital, write, read, call OA friends, and always have time to talk to them if they call me. All this from a person who, less than two months before coming to OA, spent Christmas in a wheelchair.

It's a beautiful life this Higher Power has created for us, and I for one really want to live and enjoy it.

Off in the distance sits that chocolate ship of mine. I do not have to go back to it unless I choose to. Thank God, today I have a choice.

Stick around, folks. I am going to sink the Good Ship Lollipop.

21

It Ran in the Family

WHEN I WAS SEVEN my mother nearly died and I, the oldest of three children, was "farmed out" for most of one school year. Until that time, I had been a thin, asthmatic child who didn't care about food. During my mother's illness I stayed with three different families, and I gained so much weight that when I came back home my family nicknamed me "Butterball."

I was brought up in a rural part of the Midwest that never really shook off the Depression. Bible Belt Baptists, my family on both sides could be divided into two groups: grossly overweight women who were compulsive overeaters and skinny men who were alcoholics. Naturally, I identified with the women, especially my big, diabetic grandmother whose fate I always believed I would share.

I never felt close to my mother, who couldn't show love and was constantly critical, but at thirteen I made friends with a fine, loving neighbor woman who gave me my first real feeling of acceptance. Like my relatives, she was obese.

Throughout my years at home, my mother forced me to go on unpalatable or bizarre diets to keep my weight down. I was a size 14 or 16 during most of my teen years, but she made me feel so ugly and fat that in my mind there was no difference between that size and the 26½ I was ultimately to become.

In college, I was able to keep my weight at a reasonable level until my senior year, when I had my first sexual experiences. This triggered an anxiety reaction and I went up to 180 pounds in a few months. That weight seemed the end of the world to me and, for the first time, I went on a diet voluntarily. Meantime, I stopped dating and the weight came off easily.

The next year I went to graduate school in the east. I was desperately lonely because I didn't fit in with the sophistication, and I became rather promiscuous. In one school year I went from a size 14 to a 20½ . That was the beginning of years of misery, because I never again got below that size and never again felt like a normal person until I got to Overeaters Anonymous at age thirty-five.

The intervening years were marked by depression, self-hatred, and the steady upward toll of pounds. I was in therapy for depression for at least ten years, always thinking I ate because I was depressed, not admitting to myself that the reverse was true: I was depressed because I ate. I ate on the way to therapy and I ate after therapy, and hardly ever talked about my weight or the food with any of my therapists. I would only talk about it when I was dieting, just as the only time I ever got on the scale was when I had been dieting for at least two weeks. Denial was my big defense.

The diets I tried were the same ones everyone tries. I

even had a staple in my ear once, put there by an osteopath "acupuncturist" who told me to wiggle my ear anytime I wanted to eat. Most of the time I wiggled after I ate, so it didn't do any good. I never tried diet pills. I considered myself too good and pure and drug free for that, so I just kept on drugging myself daily with sugar and gaining more weight.

I could lose 40 pounds in six weeks anytime I chose, but since that was inevitably followed by a 50-pound gain in a few months' time, I gradually gave up dieting altogether. I had become interested in astrology, and I convinced myself that my chart showed I was doomed to a lifetime of obesity.

On the surface, my life was successful. I lived in a lovely house, I was dating a beautiful, sensitive man who loved me, and I had my first book in the process of publication. I had finally arranged my career so that I could work at home most of the time, as I had always wanted to do. But I was bingeing and gaining weight, and when I topped 280, I wanted to kill myself. The last straw—or perhaps the first step toward OA— was another look at my astrology chart. It was all set up for a repeat of the conditions that had coincided with a 100-pound weight gain twelve years earlier. I was within bingeing distance of 300 pounds.

I started a last-ditch effort at dieting. I threatened myself that if it didn't work I'd have to go to Overeaters Anonymous which a friend had told me about. Strangely enough, though I loved Alcoholics Anonymous (a close friend is a recovering alcoholic, and he had taken me to a few meetings), OA sounded grim. I had been impressed with AA and had even begun to absorb some of the philosophy; still, I was sure OA couldn't do me any good.

Having flopped miserably at my "last ditch" diet, I

binged my way through one last holiday season. Early in January, I dragged myself through a snowstorm to my first OA meeting.

I was not one of those people who achieve instant abstinence. My emotional reaction in those first few weeks was like unleashing a cyclone of pain. It meant facing all the feelings I used to eat to hide, such as anger, loneliness, desire—and the way it feels to say yes to people when I really want and need to say no.

I stubbornly resisted taking a sponsor. The image of my controlling, dominating mother and her forced diets made my defiance very powerful on this point. I kept turning it over in meetings, as I was told, and gradually felt more at peace with it. It wasn't until two months into the program, when I was approaching my usual 40-pound turnaround point, that I began to see I had to take a sponsor if I wanted to keep what the program was giving me. Finally, my Higher Power got impatient with my shillyshallying and moved a fine woman who had been watching my struggles to ask if I wanted her to sponsor me. I accepted fearfully—she seemed so forbiddingly strict—and within a week I had my abstinence!

I lost weight at a dizzying pace: 110 pounds and twelve sizes in nine months. The food was comfortable most of the time—more comfortable, I had to admit, than my new body and my new identity. As much as I had fantasized about becoming a normal-size person, I was terrified when it actually happened.

Passing from a size 18 to a 16 was a real crisis; it seemed to symbolize crossing the barrier between being a freaky, fat person and joining the human race. People would say, "You must be so happy," and I couldn't honestly say yes. For about a month, I was incredibly uptight, fearful, and uncomfortable. I discovered I was afraid of men, and I also isolated myself emotionally from everyone—in program and out.

I handled this the same way I have handled each crisis I faced since joining OA. (Crises don't stop just because I'm abstinent.) I work the program twice as hard. There isn't a tool I don't use. I go to more meetings and make sure I turn over exactly what's bother bothering me. It helps. I listen at meetings as though my life depends on it—because it does. I especially listen to people with similar problems, and I home in like a laser beam on people who have relapsed, because it can happen to me if I don't learn from others' mistakes. I make phone calls. I pray for guidance. I write out my feelings and then burn what I've written. It's like burning old, self-defeating attitudes, and while they burn I pray that these attitudes will change. When I apply all aspects of the program to a crisis and trust that it is a phase rather than a life sentence, the crisis passes.

When the food thoughts come, I take them as feelings, not commands to be acted on. In fact, a little way into the program I learned that I forced food down when I didn't even want it. I often ate when I was merely thirsty. I realized that sometimes when I was binging I didn't even like the food; it became an enormous burden to consume it all. Now, I try to make mealtime serene and pleasant. I say a simple grace before each meal: "God, thank you for this beautiful food, and thank you that I don't have to eat too much of it."

I have become contented with my new body and my new identity. Now, when people say, "You must be so happy," I practically sing out that I really am. I'm still startled when I see myself in a mirror or store window, and I can still be moved to tears by a medium size that fits. I no longer have the self-loathing that comes with feeling like a freak. The male attention I am getting amazes and pleases me. I have become used to all this, but I am not complacent; just comfortable and very grateful. I have a life to look forward to instead of a living death.

In a sense, the body changes, wonderful as they are, are superficial. The most important gift of the program is a way to deal with life. People who are compulsive have learned only one response to stress: for the alcoholic the response is drink; for the overeater it is food. Whatever the stress, we ate. It didn't really help that much, but we didn't know what else to do. Now I know what to do: I work my program, and it helps in a way food never did. Not only do I feel better for the moment, but my life gets better, too. It's a wonderful feeling.

22

The Keys to Freedom

My story is a simple one. As I listen in meetings I find how much alike I am to others. This comes as a surprise because for many years I felt I was different.

My first memory is of being given food to make me feel better, and I was quite happy to get it. I taught my self to cook at an early age because my mother worked full-time and it was the only way I could get what I wanted. I badgered my parents when they wouldn't supply me, and I stole food whenever I thought I could get away with it. I had to work hard to maintain my compulsive overeating.

Because I was obese, I was teased as a child and I withdrew from people. As an only child, I found it relatively easy to become a recluse. I lived in a world of my own in which imaginary friends and television were my only companions.

In the real world I was a battered child. My parents both worked, and they had turned my care over to a maid. This woman would beat me at unpredictable times. I never told my parents because I felt that I deserved to be punished. My parents were having trouble at the time, and they often had long, bitter arguments. In my child's mind I believed these problems were my fault, so I took the beatings by the maid as a kind of penitence for all the trouble I thought I was causing.

My parents thought my bruises were the result of normal childhood accidents. When they discovered the truth, they fired the maid. But three years of physical abuse left quite an impression on me.

My self-concepts were seriously out of line. I remember when I was nine years old I went to see a great uncle whom I had never met. When he saw me, he picked me up and threw me into the air. I thought he was either God or Superman. I couldn't believe that anyone could do that. I thought I was so large, I was immovable. Like my great uncle, Overeaters Anonymous has lifted me up when I thought I was beyond help.

When I was thirteen, my parents decided it wasn't baby fat anymore and took me to a doctor for a diet. Having gotten into trouble at school, I was also taken to a psychiatrist. I lost thirty pounds on the doctor's diet by simply not eating. However, I soon became ill, and I had to eat in order to get well. I gained all the weight back—and more. I didn't think much of the diet, but I loved the cure.

The psychiatrist was just about as successful. I sat for six years in silence in her office. I trusted no one, yet I wanted desperately for her to help me. She kept telling my parents that since I refused to talk I didn't have to go back, but I continued to return. I didn't have anyplace else to go.

When I was fifteen my father, whom I worshiped, had a

nervous breakdown. He had entered the hospital a relatively young man of forty and came out three months later with gray hair, walking with a cane and looking like a man twenty years older. I grieved for him. For an entire summer I stayed in the house, going from my bedroom to the kitchen. The only time I went out was to visit the psychiatrist. My weight shot up dramatically.

The psychiatrist suggested that I would be better off somewhere else, so I went to live with my aunt and uncle. I wanted to change, but I didn't know how. My way was to go on a diet. I didn't know how much I weighed because I refused to get on a scale. After dieting for some time, I did weigh myself and found the scale registering 212. I lost another 55 pounds, but I made no other change in myself, so the weight didn't stay off.

The remainder of my high school years were filled with depression and self-imposed loneliness. I learned to live one day at a time in a negative sense. I dragged myself through each day living only for the time I could eat. During this period I came very close to committing suicide.

When I went to college, I tried to get out and be with people. I went to a girls' school and found that everybody was dieting. I made friends by going on whatever diet the other girls happened to be on. Eventually, I even began dating.

I have learned since coming to OA that whatever we turn to in times of trouble is our Higher Power. I turned to food, and when food didn't help, I turned to diets. If food wouldn't make things better, then being thin would. In college I began to diet compulsively. My weight went down, but it never stayed down for long. I wanted desperately to be like everybody else but I felt that I was so different it was impossible. I thought if

I were married, I would be normal. I wanted people to do for me what I could not do for myself.

In my senior year in college, I was faced with the prospect of going out on my own. I met a man who was willing to marry me, and within a year of that marriage I had gone up over 200 pounds and I had become a battered wife. I accepted this as a fate I deserved.

My husband hated my obesity, and I hated myself. I was not a pleasant person to be with. I tried dieting with and without pills. Nothing worked. Once, in pastoral counseling, I lost seventy-five pounds. But the counseling ended, and the diet wore out. Within six months I had regained all the weight.

I joined a commercial diet club and became a compulsive weight watcher. If the club didn't have an opinion on a topic, I didn't either. I lost the weight again over a period of two years. Finally I left because I felt there had to be more to life than weighing in every week.

My weight began to climb again. I knew I needed help but everything had failed. I had read about OA in Ann Landers' column. I believed in two things: food and Ann Landers. She had said that OA worked, so I decided to try it. There was one problem, however. I didn't know where OA was. I decided that if I ever stumbled over OA or if it ever fell on top of me, I would look into it.

A couple of months later I heard a spot announcement for OA on the radio, but I took no action. I waited a week before I called the radio station. "You don't still have the telephone number for Overeaters Anonymous, do you?" I asked. They did.

At my first meeting, I decided I didn't want to get mixed up with a bunch of religious fanatics. All I wanted was a diet, and I didn't see how God could help there. However, I believed in Ann Landers, so I kept coming back.

I thought it would be enough just to attend meetings. I tried to play my old game, which was to sit and say nothing. The people made no demands on me, though they seemed to care and some even telephoned me. However, I had a secret. They were the compulsive overeaters, not I. I knew how to lose weight. All I needed was a little group support.

For nine months I attended meetings and gained thirty-five pounds. I kept waiting for something to happen that would make me not want to eat anymore. It didn't. We were a small group and since I always came back, I was asked to get involved in service. That kept me coming back when I lost faith in Ann Landers. I also listened. I began to see that the people who were trying to make the Steps a part of their lives were changing, and good things were happening to them. I wanted that, too.

The insanity of my disease was evident to everyone but me. My life was in shambles. I had gained weight while attending meetings regularly, and I had no reason to believe that it would stop. I hated my job. I teach, and my students were noticing my weight gain. My marriage was not bliss, either. Yet I thought all I needed was a diet!

I went back to the doctor, who made it clear that he could offer me nothing new. I even returned to the diet club, but I could not sit through the lectures. In desperation, I went back into therapy. After a binge, I told the therapist about it and wanted to know what she was going to do about it. To my amazement, she said she didn't have any magic cures and that if I were truly a compulsive overeater, I'd better get back to OA and do exactly what they told me.

I had no choices left. I made a decision to test the program. I challenged this Higher Power to get me through a day of abstinence. I lived through the day, and nobody was more surprised than I was. That evening I went to a meeting and the speaker said, "When all else fails, follow directions." The directions were to get a sponsor, read the literature, use the telephone, act "as if," and use the Steps. I got a sponsor at the end of the meeting, and by the grace of God I have been abstinent from that time to this—a period of five years. I lost the forty pounds I needed to lose the first year, and I have been maintaining my normal weight since then. Before the program, I never kept weight off for more than three days.

My progress has been slow. For the first few months the food plan was my Higher Power. However, I began to turn small things over. When I had done everything I could and felt nothing worse could happen, I would turn the problem over without regard to who or what would take it. To my amazement, every time I did this something good followed. My belief that a Higher Power—God—could help me came slowly, but it came.

Step Three came when, in an effort to help someone else, I memorized the Third-Step prayer on page 63 in the "Big Book". I didn't understand it or even believe it at first, but I repeated it daily. Finally, after being abstinent for almost a year, I could feel the surrender, and it was beautiful. The longer I am in the program, the more the impact of this prayer grows and deepens within me. For the first time in my life I am free to deal with life without having to resort to the indignity of using food to get me through.

I continued in therapy, and for the first time it was working. The therapy helped me to be open to OA, and OA helped me to be open to therapy. After a year and a half of abstinence, I took my Fourth and Fifth steps with my therapist. Much to my surprise (and disappointment) she didn't turn green or faint. From this, I was able to go to people in OA and share.

I became willing to have my defects of character removed. These defects were comfortable, and I hung onto them dearly. I never knew it was okay to be happy. Someone had to tell me. The old comfortable, familiar pain has gradually given way to peace. I am not perfect, but I have been granted the gifts of change and growth. I know now that with the help of my Higher Power I am no longer locked into a prison of unhappy ways. The program has given me the keys to freedom.

I have learned two important things. One is that life may bring pleasure or it may bring pain, but the program has given me the tools to deal with whatever comes. I have also learned that life is to be enjoyed. I spend time in meetings and doing Twelfth-Step work which brings me both peace and joy. And I am able to go out into the world and be at peace there, too.

23 ————————

Journey Through Deception

BEFORE I CAME THROUGH the OA door five years ago, I had done little about my weight problem. I blamed my sluggish metabolism. I complained that other people could eat more than I did without gaining a pound. Life was so unfair!

Years ago I discovered that when I kept busy, the weight melted off without any conscious effort on my part. So I started a cycle that alternated between distraction and depression for the next twenty years. While busy, I maintained a low weight of 120 pounds. When the distraction lost its charm, as it inevitably did, I became depressed and immobilized. My weight would skyrocket, rising higher with each slump.

At five-feet, three inches, I weighed 178 pounds. I know this only because I visited a diet club where they weighed me. Normally I shunned scales, mirrors, and cameras so that I could keep my self-deceptions intact. I went through my fat periods in a state of isolation and suspension, waiting till I could become "real" again with another spate of activity.

Five years ago I was in another slump. This time I could not afford to wait for something to spur me out of it. I was facing possible bankruptcy and had two lawsuits pending. It might be years before these were settled. I had to come to terms with my weight problem now. I had no experience with other diet systems, but the choice was easy: I was broke and OA was free.

From the time of my first meeting I abstained and called my food in daily to the sponsor I chose that night. The food plan I adopted was a new game to me and by playing it I lost 52 pounds in four and a half months. My "tools" were diet pop, artificial sweeteners, and nail biting. I went to many meetings but treated them as living soap operas. I tuned out what I thought of as the "religious" part of the program. I stayed aloof because I did not want to identify with losers, i.e., compulsive overeaters. I was there to lose weight, not to change my personality or get religion. I thought my personality was just fine, and I already believed in a loving God. When my weight got down to 120 pounds, I left OA with my slim body and my fat head.

I continued to abstain by myself and lost four more pounds. I was filled with complacence: I had the magic formula and I could do it alone! For the next two and a half years I weighed myself daily, kept a log of everything I ate and "passed" as a thin person. Certainly, I never gave any credit to OA.

I did learn three things from that first experience with OA: to follow a food plan, to be aware of what I ate, and never to overeat because of guilt about overeating. I applied the discipline I had learned from abstinence to other areas of my life and was quite successful. My new job was the best I had ever had. I learned sports and tried my hand at new hobbies such as dressmaking. Every relationship in my life bloomed. I never looked or felt better.

But something was missing. Toward the end of this period my weight began to climb until it reached 142 pounds. The new pants I had just made soon would not fit.

Back I came to OA, more desperate, less cocky, more willing. While I had been away I had given up my "tools." I decided not to take them back. This time I would be forced to work the program instead of transferring my compulsions. This time, if I blew it, I knew it would be with food.

I began by attacking my self-serving deceptions.

I had no metabolism problem. My glands worked just as well at one weight as another. I couldn't blame heredity. True, my mother and sisters were compulsive overeaters, but my father always ate moderately and kept his normal weight.

I couldn't blame my attitudes toward food on my conditioning. My mother had served large portions and insisted that I finish them. But millions of youngsters are given too much to eat and are urged to finish it because "wasting food is a sin," yet they do not wind up gorging themselves. It was true that it pleased my mother to see me enjoy her cooking. But I rebelled against her authority in other ways constantly and felt no compunction about not pleasing her.

It had not been my parents who told me to devour my lunch on the way to school, to steal candy from neighbors, to take nickels from my mother's purse for candy bars. They told me candy was junk and stealing was wrong.

I could not blame lack of parental love either. I assumed

guilt by association when my mother told me that my birth coincided with her goiter operation, which left an ugly scar. I believed myself rejected when my father said that before my birth he was fearful about the Depression and really didn't want another child. I took up martyrdom because my parents gave me approval only when I was polite and obedient, and they seemed unable to accept my feelings.

But I came to realize that most people are raised with conditional love; that nearly everyone is sometimes made to feel inferior by his parents; that many men and women lack self-worth. But they do not become overeaters. While I cleared my head of these old tapes, I had to abstain.

I could not blame my compulsion on the burdens I had grown up with. I was born with some physical abnormalities. My mother and sister were psychotic. My brother was mentally retarded. My father deserted his family when I was twelve, and we were destitute. We lived in a slum where violence was commonplace. Food was my bit of sweetness in such misery.

But I have learned to live with each of these facts, and I have grown stronger because of them. Others have just as much to contend with and they do not choose to eat over it. Living in the past, bemoaning my fate is just a way to justify my eating.

I have learned to see myself as one of God's children, neither the best nor the worst. I know I have talent, intelligence and ability, and I have had many fine accomplishments. But my self-worth is not validated by any of these. I can love and accept my weaknesses as well as my strengths because they are part of me. I make many mistakes as I reach toward growth, but I no longer expect perfection from myself or anyone else.

Despite this acceptance, I am still tempted at times to kill myself by overeating. My loving self has to work a very tough program to prevent my destroying self from taking over.

I have learned to value more of the simple things, such as the sheer joy of being alive. My happiness depends on my attitude, not on circumstances. Whether I am a compulsive overeater or not, life presents daily problems; how happy I want to be while dealing with them is up to me.

I know now that my immature personality was the root of my problem and that growing up was the solution. I learned to accept my feelings and to take responsibility for channeling them constructively. I went through the Steps. I became more patient, compassionate, and honest. The changes in me brought loving responses from those around me. My weight dropped to 105 pounds.

But I had more to learn. It was painful to realize that my feelings were not the cause of my eating. I had gone through temper tantrums, guilt, loneliness, resentment, fear—many negative emotions—all my life. I overate not because of the feelings, but because I was food-obsessed and I gave myself license to overeat by producing the negative emotions. In other words, I made myself upset so that I had an excuse to overeat.

I may never be emotionally mature. This is an endless journey. But while I travel on it, I cannot use my lack of maturity to justify my eating. Emotional and physical binges are no longer substitutes for action.

I see now that the alternative to abstinence, for me, is suicide. I am no longer able to tell myself lies to excuse binges. In order to abstain, I keep these things in mind: (1) I believe, for today, that I must compensate for my lack of food brakes by maintaining those disciplines that enable me to be moderate. (2) For me, one bite of certain carbohydrates is suicide, fast or slow, because I lack psychosomatic immunity to them. (3) I cannot indulge in negativity, because it blocks out my program awareness. Self-pity is a luxury I cannot afford because it causes amnesia, and I revert to old habits. (4) My primary responsibility is to abstain. All roles—wife, mother, friend, employee—come second. If abstinence is not first, I will lose it. Everything that interferes with it must go. (5) I never have it made. My compulsion never goes away; it waits for me to become careless or cocky. (6) The OA program at its toughest is better than bingeing. Life at its dreariest or scariest is better than death by overeating.

I am continuing to discard more lies. I have the love of OA friends and my family in making this painful, joyous journey. I am grateful because I know that getting rid of deceptions makes me freer to see the ones that still blind me, still bind me.

24

Fat Is Not My Destiny

Food was a family affair. My brothers and I were born in the years following World War II and we were caught up in the race for affluence and security, one symbol of which was unlimited food. Any occasion called for a feast: birthdays, holidays, vacations, Sunday excursions, births, deaths, weddings, reunions. Once the basic overeating pattern was established, I elaborated on it. No matter where I went to school there was always a store or pastry shop or candy counter I could patronize, and I resorted to stealing nickels and dimes and quarters from my father's change box to supplement my inadequate allowance.

At home I ate anything I could get my hands on, straight from the box, can or jar, cooked or uncooked, baked or unbaked; it made no difference. I had no discriminating tastes. Canned spaghetti tasted as delicious to me as any treasured Italian family recipe. I couldn't even appreciate my

German grandmother's baking as any better than Sara Lee's. I lost babysitting jobs because I ate everything except the baby.

My compulsive overeating may have had something to do with my older brother's chronic illness. He spent his entire childhood in and out of hospitals and my parents were preoccupied with his health. Just as his disease was brought under control and I was struggling through adolescence, my younger brother developed schizophrenia, and my parents' concern shifted to him. Somehow, in the midst of all this, food became my reward and punishment, love and companionship.

By the time I was in high school, I weighed 150 pounds, a weight below which I have never fallen in my adult life. I carried it well—in the same place a barrel does—and the straight skirts, tucked-in blouses and belted shirtwaists then in fashion made it impossible to disguise.

I never dated, and I quickly resigned myself to cutting remarks and snickers when my stomach growled in class. I eventually kept mostly to myself to avoid getting hurt, and I convinced myself that this was the way I wanted it.

After graduating from college, I became a high school librarian in a small school. I moved in with two college friends who were also teaching there and was ready to believe I had it made for the rest of my life. During the second year, reality set in and teaching became a serious business. Soon it deteriorated into a battle. My first major disappointment was the realization that I was not going to make it in the profession. I didn't see the pattern building until it was too late, but that failure made me resentful and angry. I was angry at the kids because in spite of my best efforts to direct and control their lives, they failed me and that reflected on me. I was angry at the principal, whom I considered incompetent; I was angry at the other teachers who seemed successful; I was angry at my parents because I believed they had pressured me into teaching; and I was angry at myself for letting things get out of control, including my weight which had gone up thirty-eight pounds in four years.

I fought it every way I could, from letters to Dear Abby to psychiatric counseling, from memberships in health spas and diet clubs to books on losing weight. Nothing worked. Everything emphasized food. I was still looking forward to eleven o'clock for the celery sticks, counting the minutes until I could eat the apple I had saved from lunch, planning menus and substitutions that read like computer printouts. As an example of my obsessiveness, I had by that time collected forty-three cookbooks and nine shoeboxes of clipped recipes. (You won't find this food emphasis in OA. The emphasis is on you and me and us as people, not on food.) The amazing thing about this most important time in my life is that through it all I never even knew I was angry. I mean, after all, everybody else was failing me; it was their fault, not mine. Lord knows I was trying. Outwardly, I was controlled, calm, in command. Inwardly, the growing anger was eating me up, and I was trying to stop it with food.

It was inevitable that a crisis would occur with such pressures building, and in my fifth and final year of teaching it did. I almost killed a student in one blinding moment of anger that broke through. In February of that year, I was on hall duty and enduring the usual hassles that go with the job. That particular day Tommy Troublemaker chose to make himself unbearable. I had just shooed him down the stairs for the third time, then stepped into a teacher's room. She was the play director and she showed me some of the props her peo-

Fat Is Not My Destiny

ple had been collecting, one of which was a heavy iron crowbar. I was standing by her desk talking, my hand on that crowbar, when Tommy sauntered through the door with some smart remark. In a flash of anger, my hand closed around the crowbar and raised it. Had the teacher not grabbed my wrist, I probably would have taken Tommy's head off, although I can't be sure of that.

I laid the crowbar back on the desk and went to the superintendent's office, where I wrote out my resignation on the back of a lunch menu and turned it in. For the three months remaining in the school year, that woman and two other good friends ran interference for me, and there were no further incidents. But I lived in fear of what might happen and in agony over what I had found out about myself.

When school was over, I moved out of the state with the sole intention of vegetating for a year and bringing myself and my weight under control. Actually, I wasn't moving to a place so much as I was moving away from people and things. Among them was a man who wanted to marry me; I thought there must be something wrong with him if he could love me.

The most joyous discovery I made upon my arrival in my new community was supermarkets that were open twenty-four hours a day. I spent my first three weeks eating and watching television, crying, depressed. I never got dressed except to go out and buy food. For the first time in my life I knew what real loneliness was.

I began going to OA meetings soon after I got settled, but my first weeks with the program were exasperating. I was disagreeable, hostile and resentful that I had to be there at all. But mostly I was frightened that if I tried to follow the program and failed, there was nothing left. Also, I am agnostic and my first impression was that I had happened upon a group of evangelists who would attempt to convince me that nothing could happen until I accepted their God. They quickly disproved that. Once I stopped looking for flaws and began listening in earnest, I was able to find a Higher Power that works for me. My Higher Power is the group, the people, my friends.

Abstinence and weight loss came only after I accepted the fact that this program is something I cannot manage alone; I need all the help I can get, and there's no shame in that.

Many other physical symptoms of overeating have disappeared. Gone are dry skin, joint pains, sinusitis, headaches. I'm off thyroid after twenty-two years. I can cross my legs under a table without causing a commotion. My knee socks come up to my knees now. These are measurements that make me feel good about myself.

Emotionally I am freer, and spiritually I am at peace with myself and with my Higher Power. The quality of my life is improving every day.

My salvation, if you will, came with the realization that being fat is not in my mind or my destiny, but is rather a symptom of a disease, compulsive overeating. Thanks to an incident that occurred during my first year in the program, I know that compulsive overeating is controllable, but not curable.

On that particular occasion, shortly before Christmas, I led an OA meeting during which I told the group that I was to be married—to the same man I had moved away from. I was feeling worthy for the first time in my life—open and loving. I flew to my parents' home the next day for a long weekend and felt very proud of the way I resisted temptation and handled my food while there, because Christmas at home is a feast from beginning to end. I also dealt with my family's rather hostile reaction to my marriage plans in what I considered a calm, adult manner. I even smiled benignly during all the hassles of holiday travel and returned home ready to begin a new year.

The next day I went to work and someone opened a box of chocolates. Within two hours I had eaten the entire thing, and it was supposed to have been shared among five people. I didn't feel the least bit guilty about it. After work, I drove to a mall and bought my favorite binge foods. As an example of the extremes to which compulsive overeaters are driven, I was too ashamed to eat these things in public and couldn't wait to get home, so in nine-degree weather in a car with no heat, I sat in the parking lot and ate the stuff with my gloves on and darn near froze to death.

Then I realized that within a short span of time, I was back to square one and doing the disgusting, revolting things I hated, and what was there to eat about anyway? I was happier than I had ever been in my life. I was to be married to someone I loved very much. My work was going well. I got A's in my semester course work. I had many friends. My future was bright. Why did I feel the need to punish myself this way?

I had no answer. I still don't, but that's not what matters. What matters is that I started the car and got to an OA meeting where I shared what I had just done.

OA people don't judge or react with horror when they hear something like that. They listen, they talk, they suggest readings, they call me later to see how I'm doing, they stop in the middle of their day when I call to talk. With this help and encouragement, I was able to break the vicious rationalization that because I did it once, another time won't hurt, or I'll wait until January 1st and start all over again, I started again right then, and although the compulsive feeling didn't leave me for days, I didn't eat about it. And soon I was okay.

But I got a good dose of humility which I badly needed, and the complacency I was beginning to feel was gone permanently. I know now that this job is never done. But I take it a day at a time, twelve hours at a time, sometimes fifteen minutes at a time, and that's the way I win.

25

Beautiful Woman Inside and Out

HOW DOES ONE TELL in a few pages the story of fifteen and a half years in Overeaters Anonymous? How can I describe in a limited number of words what seven years of abstinence means coming after eight years of alternating between defiance, despair, and submission to the program? How do I tell you of the gratitude in my heart for the miracles of abundance, joy, health, strength, and power in my life today? Mine was a life lived in insecurity, self-doubt, chronic illness, addiction, and obesity.

When people look at me today, they see a tall, attractive, slender woman. There seems to be a quality about me that many call "beautiful." It is not my outward appearance, but rather something from within that comes from living the Twelve Steps to the best of my ability. I could not have imagined such a gift. When I daydreamed or "prayed," it was to be thin magically and to have Prince Charming find me. I prayed for the money to pay my bills, take a trip, buy a new car, and so on. Who would have thought to pray for a fullness from within that can make a spastic colon behave normally, control the chronic leg cramps and backaches and palpitations, and take away the desire for refined sugar and flour? That would be asking for miracles

All I wanted was a nice house, a good school for my children, two cars in the garage, and that I should look good on Saturday night. By praying for specific things, I was limiting the good in my life and expanding and giving power to negativity. It took many years to understand this; the gift of "life while living" came hard for me.

For years I tried frantically to prove that after I got thin I could eat anything I wanted anytime I wanted it. Always, I regained the lost weight, plus a few pounds, never being able to wear the same clothes from one season to another, always on a diet, whether eating or starving. I have known the pain and humiliation of not being able to participate in sports and of being laughed at by the other kids as well as by teachers, store clerks, strangers, and even friends. Though my recovery is not unique in Overeaters Anonymous, it may help the reader's understanding to know the specific ills from which I have recovered. To the best of my recollection, they are: food obsession, the weight yo-yo syndrome, the scale running my life, my size being my self-worth, living on fifteen pills a day (amphetamines, diuretics, laxatives), smoking three packs of cigarettes a day, drinking ten to fifteen cans of diet soda a day, drinking fifteen mugs of coffee a day, chewing three packs of sugarless gum a day, chronic leg cramps, chronic lower backaches, chronic need for excessive sleep, spastic colon.

These symptoms were a way of life for me. I believed and

trusted them. They kept me guilty and failing and never achieving the good within me. While I can say that I have experienced moments of great sensual pleasure, the deep fear within me always brought me crashing to new lows. It was a price I expected to pay for grabbing and snatching at material things.

My race for possessions and sensual gratification gave me a good deal of fun and enjoyment, which is recorded with love in my memory. But the price I had to pay in self-hate, rage at my children, and poor health (I never really felt well unless I was using a substance or making love) was too high.

And one day it stopped. I don't know when or how it stopped. It happened in stages, inch by inch, pound by pound. One day, after two and a half years of rigid abstinence and fear of food, I woke up and understood that I no longer had to fear sugar and flour. I know neither the time nor the process by which these dependencies were removed. I know only that when I stopped trying to control the timetable for removal of my addictions, they were removed.

Today I celebrate seven years of abstinence, accumulated by the grace of God, one day at a time. What does that mean to me? I have come to understand that we in OA cannot have the perfect, absolute abstinence that is common to AAers. Abstinence must be a different thing for each of us. Mine is always changing and growing, just as I change and grow to meet the world and God.

What worked for me in the beginning of my OA years is no longer valid. I had to learn that strict adherence to any food plan was madness for me if I hoped to thrive in the mainstream of life.

Today I am so filled with love and gratitude for my understanding of abstinence that I find it difficult to describe. I believe abstinence can be anything we want it to be, so long as we are honest with ourselves.

I have come to know my body inside and out, better than any doctor could know it. I have not been ill in seven years except for one brief bout with flu and a minor cold. Of course, I still go for medical checkups, and I do not discount the value of medical science.

Today I am maintaining a sixty-pound weight loss in the program. The Twelve Steps are a way of life for me, reaching into every aspect of my affairs. One year ago, my husband came to the program after fighting it for nine years. He has just completed his first year of abstinence and a sixty-pound weight loss. My daughter is now in OA and actively participating in our teen program. It is a miracle in our lives and we are grateful for the abundance that has been given us.

Today I know that I have an addictive personality and that from time to time my illness will flare up. That doesn't mean I am a failure. It means I can be restored to sanity any time I choose the power. While food is no longer a problem and many outer manifestations have been removed, the illness still creeps up in emotional storms and maladjustments. That is the nature of life, and I grow from working through each experience.

There are many things that are "right" with me today, starting with the Higher Power that is at work in my life. It is a power that is within me, the highest self I can be, whom I choose to call God. God in my life is expressed through many channels, and I have a receiver that is turned on, thanks to the program. Some of the channels through which I receive God are music, poetry, literature, art, dance, people, nature, forces for good in the universe, and love. Love is surely an expression of a Higher Power in my life. Today I can give and receive love—and know that, by the grace of God, I am a beautiful woman inside and out.

26 _____

The Overachiever
Who Overcame

DURING MY SCHOOL YEARS I learned that I could get approval from my parents by being a good girl and doing well academically. I brought home good report cards, and my parents were very pleased with my achievement, but I felt an emptiness that only food seemed to fill. My family did not openly display affection, and I longed for the kind of love that I saw expressed with hugs and kisses in other families.

When I realized the impossibility of losing weight, a sort of resignation set in. I accepted what the doctor told me: I would probably lose a day from my life span for every day I overate. Life seemed less worth living, anyway; I didn't care.

After my freshman year in college, I spent a summer in volunteer service at the National Institute of Health in Bethesda, Maryland. As a "normal" control subject in medical research, I requested a moderate diet in the hospital, and my weight dropped from 200 pounds to 170 in thirty days. This proved one thing to me: I had no metabolic disorder; I was fat because I ate too much.

I came home thinner than I had ever been in my adult life and told my story of humanitarian service to a college-age church group. The idealistic president of the club was very taken with me, and we were married a few months later. I was determined to continue with college and also worked full time until our first child came two and a half years later. I was still in the superachiever syndrome. I overcompensated in the intellectual areas for my painful and overwhelming deficiencies in nearly every other area of my life.

My eating was out of control. I gained weight with both my pregnancies, especially during the six months following delivery. I was totally unable to cope with the housework and we lived in filth and clutter. The children were colicky and drove me up the wall. My husband was progressing down the road of alcoholism, and sex had become very distasteful to me. I went once or twice a week to a family therapist for three years during the early part of our marriage. I appreciated the therapist's love and caring, and I became dependent on her. But I was unable to overcome my sloth, sexual aversion, binge eating, and inability to cope with my children.

After eight years, I got my college degree and went to work. It was hard to find a job at 215 pounds, even with my honors in mathematics. I liked to pretend my difficulty was due to discrimination against women, but actually I was uninsurable under many company insurance plans, and some employers had to turn me down. The job I finally got served two main purposes: it kept me from eating for eight hours, since I was a secret eater; and it filled an ego need. I could do well at work and pay someone else to clean my house and take care of the children.

By the time I was twenty-nine, I had eaten my way to 240 pounds and developed the symptoms of diabetes. Again a doctor gave me a frightening talk on the danger to my life and health, and this time I followed his diet to the letter—for a period of five months and a weight loss of 50 pounds. At 190 my diabetic symptoms disappeared, and so did my will power. Again my eating was out of control, and I began vomiting after my binges to keep from regaining the weight.

Realizing the seriousness of trying to control my weight by vomiting, I went to a diet club. I lost 20 pounds in sixteen weeks and received my gold pin while bingeing on enormous quantities of "free" foods. After that I couldn't limit my binges to the low carbohydrate vegetables. As soon as I had one slice of bread too much, I knew I would eat the whole loaf because it would have to come up anyway. before finding OA, I spent a full year bingeing and regurgitating daily while faithfully attending my diet club meetings, trying all their new recipes, and not losing another pound.

Then, after twelve years of an increasingly rocky marriage, I filed for divorce. In desperation, my husband went to Alcoholics Anonymous and—miracle of miracles—he got sober. I was directed to Al-Anon where I saw firsthand the beautiful changes in family members who practiced AA's Twelve Steps in their own lives. My husband and I decided to give the marriage another chance.

Strangely, my bingeing rapidly got worse, and my life became even more unmanageable. An Al-Anon friend directed me to OA. She told me that with my compulsion I stood about as much chance of success in Al-Anon as my alcoholic husband would. A compulsive overeater can't fully grasp and develop a spiritual way of life while bingeing, any more than an alcoholic can while still drinking. To be honest with Step Three, I could only say I would turn over my will and my life except in the area of food. I read the OA pamphlet with the fifteen questions, and I knew without a doubt that I was a compulsive overeater.

I hardly dared hope that OA could solve my various living problems, as it so obviously had for many who spoke at my first meeting. I would be content if only I could stop destroying myself with food. I desperately needed and wanted what those OAers had, so I did as they suggested and took a sponsor the first night. She said, "If you want what I have, do what I did." She had lost 130 pounds by abstaining and diligently following the Twelve Steps.

I had proved I couldn't do it my way before I came to OA. Now I needed to be open and receptive to the discipline in eating and in the other areas of my life which were suggested in OA. I somehow managed to abstain, one day at a time. I held on to the idea that I just had to postpone eating more until the next mealtime. I read the OA pamphlet, "Before You Take That First Compulsive Bite," with every meal, and I realized that I wanted and needed abstinence more than I wanted and needed food. I quit fighting, and I sensed for the first time in my life a real freedom from the self-destructive urge to overeat.

It was a relief to know that I didn't have to subscribe to any particular belief or faith in order to get on with the steps. I called myself an agnostic, but I knew that the OA group was a power greater than myself, that the Twelve Steps were a better way to live than I could ever devise, and that God for me was beyond understanding.

Gradually, I became free of the bonds of the past and

willing to try to set right those things that I could. Every day of continued abstinence became an amends to my body for the abuse of overeating in the past. I began to overcome my sloth by doing a number of things every day which I didn't want to do: making my bed, doing the dishes, brushing my teeth, and taking a shower. After a time, these tasks became a part of the disciplined way of life which, along with my abstinence, led me to sanity.

The sexual problem in my marriage was overcome as I practiced the Third-Step prayer given in the "Big Book" of Alcoholics Anonymous. I was released in a large measure from the bondage of self: self-consciousness, self-centeredness, and selfishness.

I treated sex in my inventory as suggested in Chapter Five of the "Big Book." I came to realize that the most serious offense I committed was the deliberate interference with the development of love and withholding its expression. Overcoming the frigidity in my marriage and clearing away the blocks to the expression of love for my children, family, and others were the most profound changes I experienced in OA, aside from the changes in my eating habits.

After eight months of abstinence I had the first of several deeply moving experiences which indicated the presence of a power that was doing for me what I couldn't do for myself. I began to call that power God. I had visited a dear OA friend who had broken her long term abstinence after surgery. She would have given anything to move the clock back. As I drove to work the next morning, I thought of the many who had come to OA before me and after me who were losing their abstinence, and I wondered when it would be my turn, since I was no better than they were. Then it dawned on me that of course I was no better. I was utterly powerless. And yet I had been abstaining for eight months. How did I do it? I didn't do it. A power greater than myself whose presence I felt at that moment was doing it through me. I could accept that gift for today. And there was no reason to doubt that the gift of abstinence would continue to be available on a daily basis. Only my self-will, my decision to eat, could take it away from me. In acknowledging my true source, I lost my fear and became responsible for myself.

I'm grateful that I have the disease of compulsive overeating, because it turned my life around and transported me to a higher plane. The illness that was killing me is now my chief asset.

27

The Athiest Who Made a Zif

A COMPULSIVE EATER, they say, is a sort of guilt detector. If there's any guilt around, you pick it up, take it home, nurture it, feed it, love it.

I felt guilty as a kid because I used to have nightmares all the time. They were always the same. Some devil or monster was chasing me, and I'd wake up screaming. This happened when I was about ten years old. In that same year, I figured out a way to get rid of these dreams. I became an atheist. Since there was no God, He wasn't going to send devils or monsters after me.

I stopped having the nightmares. I would say, "Go ahead, throw a lightning bolt at me. I know you're not there. It's all those weak people who need to believe in God. Me, I'm strong. I don't need you."

What I did need was to eat and eat. At thirteen, when all the other boys were starting to go out with girls, I weighed 200 pounds. My parents took me to a doctor who gave me thyroid, which was what they used before speed was invented. When I was twenty, they found another doctor. This one put me on a "modified fast" diet. I ate nothing for two weeks at a time. This had a profound effect on me because I soon discovered that breaking such a long fast made me vomit. My stomach couldn't tolerate the food. But if I stopped every five or ten minutes on the way home, I could eat for seventy two hours straight. That really sharpened my ability to binge. In spite of the bingeing, however, I lost about 82 pounds that summer. I was down to a trim 217. It was the first time in my life that I could walk into a real people's store instead of a fat men's store where you pay twice as much for styles that went out thirty years ago. The suit I bought was olive green. I felt so good when I tried it on and it fit. It was the biggest size they had in the store, but it was a "regular" store and the suit fit.

I went back to school and decided it was time to start going out. I had never been on a date in my life. I took one girl out and the highlight of the evening was when she got out of the car. I thought, "Thank God, that's over with." I had been very uncomfortable. I didn't know what to do or say. I forced myself to try it again and it was the same: the best part of the evening was when the girl left.

At that time I was living with three roommates. One of them introduced me to a friend of a friend, a girl who was also "people." She used to come over and we'd talk. I started going out with her. We went together for about two months and finally, at twenty-one, I had sex for the first time. We got married in June. I weighed 297 pounds. I hadn't had a chance to wear that olive green suit a half dozen times before it didn't fit any more. I certainly didn't wear it at my wedding; it wouldn't have fit on one leg.

We moved to California and my life took on some really exciting aspects. I would have a giant breakfast, then go to work. At about nine-thirty the coffee shop downstairs would send up "refreshments" for the coffee break. I always had a couple. First, though, I'd sneak downstairs and have a few early ones, and after the coffee break I'd go back down and finish off what was left. Around noon, the catering truck came and I'd have a big lunch, then eat some more at the afternoon coffee break. And always, on the way home from work, I had to stop for something to eat. In the evening, after a big dinner, I would lie on the couch and watch television while my wife fed me sugar. Each night I faded into a stupor and then got up the next morning and started again.

That was the way I maintained 325 pounds. One day I walked into a drugstore and noticed a little diet book. I bought it and counted my calories for about nine months. I lost 120 pounds. Now came the ego. You see, I had always thought I was great, even when my self-worth was nonexistent. I could never admit that I was wrong. I made up "facts" to win an argument. Now, having lost that weight, I knew I was great. For one thing, when I was fat it was clear to me that I was crazy: one look told me that. But when I lost the weight, I thought I was sane because I believed it was the fat that had been making me crazy.

There's nothing more dangerous than a crazy person who thinks he's sane. I got divorced. Then I went on a spree to try to make up for all the fun I had missed. I was "going steady" with three women at the same time once, and my roommate had a list of who to tell what when they called.

I have a theory that if a person has a fat head and a thin

body, one has to catch up with the other. I maintained my weight for a while with "sensible" eating techniques such as nothing but carrots for a week. Or all the celery you can eat with nothing in between. For bingeing between fasts, laxatives were my bag. The only problem was they didn't work; I ate again as soon as I had that nice empty feeling.

Slowly, the weight started to creep up. During this second thin period, I had taken up sports. I was the fellow whose worst subject in school was gym. I would wash the coach's car, clean his desk, do anything I had to do to get out of gym. I couldn't do a single sit-up or pushup; I couldn't run thirty feet. My body was a total handicap. Now, when I lost all that weight and started surfing and playing volleyball and water skiing, it was as if I had been a quadriplegic all my life and suddenly I had full use of my limbs. My body was functioning. My body could bring me joy. It was a wonderful feeling.

But I started to gain the weight back. First slowly, then faster. I was losing my body again. There wasn't a water ski big enough to float me anymore; and snow skiing, I looked like an avalanche rolling down the hill. Nobody would play volleyball with me. I had an eleven-foot surfboard and I couldn't get out of the water on it. I had one girlfriend left, and the relationship was very tenuous. At work, where I held a technical sales position, my bosses were telling me that I was not a fit representative for the company.

One night, I lay on my bed with a pain in my chest. I knew what it was. The doctors had all promised me a heart attack by the time I was thirty. All my life I knew that was what I was going to get for my birthday unless I lost weight. In the morning, I walked across the street to the emergency room of the hospital and checked myself in. They ran an EKG, and when the orderly came out later I asked, "What is it?" He told me it was "pudgy pain."

I was an atheist; I couldn't make a solemn oath to God, but I made one to myself. This was it. I had dieted before, and I was going to do it again. It was the shortest diet I was ever on. It lasted four lanes. I walked back across the street and ate sugar for about four hours. Then I went on a diet and lost thirty-five pounds in eight weeks, and after that I went on another diet and lost twenty-five pounds in six weeks. I always gained back that weight with a little bonus—five or ten pounds for trying.

The night I hit bottom is very clear in my memory. My roommate was home. This guy was the greatest ladies' man in all of Southern California. He would go out to a bar or someplace and come home with a beautiful woman every night. That night he had come in with a girl, and I could hear them talking upstairs. I was sitting on my bed with my package of goodies next to me, eating and crying. I thought, "There's no sense trying to quit eating because I can't. For some reason I'm different from other people. The only choice I have is to just enjoy my food. I'm going to lose my job, and I'm going to die, but hopefully when I go it'll be fast; I won't have to be an invalid."

I had never heard of the Twelve Steps, and I knew nothing about Alcoholics Anonymous, but that night I took Step One. I admitted that I was powerless over food and my life was unmanageable, right at gut level. And I also took Step Three, in a way. I made a decision right then and there to turn my will and my life over to my Higher Power, which was food. But it was a good start. It set the stage.

At this time, I was being treated by my doctor for dysentery. That good man had been delighted to see me lose weight, and now he was horrified that I was gaining it all back. The dysentery I was suffering was so severe I would almost pass out. Yet I gained fourteen pounds in one month. We didn't know what caused the dysentery until after I got into Overeaters Anonymous. It was from pouring sugar into myself at such a rate that my system wouldn't tolerate it.

On one visit, the doctor ran an EKG and a heart vector. He told me things were not good. "You can't afford to gain any more weight," he said. "You have to lose it, or you're going to die."

"I know that," I said, "but don't bother to give me a diet because it's a waste of your paper."

"When you go outside," he said, "I want you to ask my secretary for the OA phone number. I have a patient who is a member and she said to have people like you call her."

A woman answered the phone. "I want you to tell me all there is to know about this Overeaters Anonymous," I told her.

"I can't do that," she said. "It's too complicated to explain."

I really believe that God put this woman there because if she had tried to tell me what Overeaters Anonymous was about, I would have said, "Phtt," and gone out and died. Instead, I went to a meeting. I sat in the back row behind a post. Two large women sat down on either side of me. I couldn't get out.

When the meeting started, the first thing I heard was "God." I thought, Hah! Now I know. The next thing, they're going to want to convert me and they're going to bless me and dip me in water. I see what the gimmick is now.

When they called the coffee break, I saw my chance. I got up and started to leave. But people flocked around me and started talking to me. It seemed I was the only newcomer there. Before I could escape, the meeting started again. The speaker started off by saying, "I used to be 325 pounds and I'm now 180 pounds and my goal is to be half the man I once was."

I thought, "Uh-huh." Then he passed his picture around and it didn't look as though it was touched up. It was a real snapshot. I didn't hear anything else that night, but after the meeting I had to talk to that man. I had to know the secret. I had to make sure he was real. He invited me to go to coffee with the group.

"No, I can't," I said. "I'm busy. Winchell's will close in three hours."

But they kept asking me and it appeared obvious that they really wanted me. No one had wanted me for anything in so long that I went.

At home, I began thinking: The speaker was thin, and she used to be fat, too. Maybe I'd better get a sponsor. I realized that I had only one telephone number—the woman I had first talked with. When I called and asked her to be my sponsor, she said, "I'd love to."

I called her every day for five months,and I got to love that lady. She was about sixty-two years old and six-foot, three-inches tall, and she talked like a truck driver. I didn't try to con her, ever. She said, "Do it," and I did it.

My Higher Power began evolving the day I heard some-one suggest that nonbelievers make "a zif." I was an atheist, not an agnostic. An agnostic has doubts. I had never doubted anything. I knew there was no God. When I learned that "a zif" meant "acting as if," I was told that I didn't have to believe in anything. All I had to do was say, "God, I don't believe you're there, but anyway, I'd like such and such."

"You're asking me to be a hypocrite," I said.

"Oh, heaven forbid! You could be a glutton, a thief and an egomaniac—vicious in every possible way; you could smell bad, you could look bad, but by God, we don't want you to be a hypocrite!"

I said, "Okay, I'll try it."

At first my Higher Power looked like my sponsor. Then he looked like me. Then, like a kind old man with a big beard. My Higher Power has always been a loving Higher Power. My sponsor told me, "You can choose anything you want, but it's got to be benevolent, not malevolent." So I started to develop a Higher Power that was sort of a spirit of the universe, and if I was in touch with that flow then I would go the easy way and good things would happen. And they did. Things just happened, one right after another. Beautiful things.

One morning I was eating breakfast and reading my twenty-four hour book when there was an earthquake. The house was rocking back and forth, and I felt a great rush of warmth several times. It was as if God was in me. He was rocking me back and forth in His arms and I was smiling. Nobody smiles during an earthquake. I sat there at the table and I picked up the twenty-four hour book and opened it and it said, "Fear not fire or earthquake." A cold chill shot through me, and I went upstairs and took a shower with one eye open, thinking, "God, please don't be standing there when I get out of this shower because I'll die. You're not supposed to be there."

It got so I was praying for parking places and getting them.

About nine months ago, I was standing in my kitchen and I felt the warm flash again. I'm happy to say it's back. I have a good conscious contact with my Higher Power. We talk to each other. He knows I'm a screw-up, that I do things wrong. But He doesn't mind. He loves me pure and true, as only a perfect being can love. I can't love you that way, and you can't love me that way because we're not perfect. Only He can love us that way.

28 ─────────

Indian Summer

LOVE AND FEAR HAVE been at war in me since I can first remember. I was the baby of the family. To me, this meant that father, mother, grandmother, three older brothers, and a big sister were all there to tell me what to do. If I tried to participate in family affairs, someone was sure to tell me to sit down, be quiet, don't show off because you don't know anything about it.

I believed them.

My parents thought that praise made children vain. Good grades in school were noted without comment. When I won a spelling contest, strangers congratulated me, but at home nothing was said. I concluded that my family did not care, that to them I was still stupid.

No one deliberately taught me these things. They are what I learned.

My older sister, who was twice my size, dominated me

completely. She was fat, poor child, and she passed her discontent on to me by convincing me that I was not only stupid but ugly. She ordered me to wait on her like a little slave. If I protested, my mother always made me surrender because she dreaded her older daughter's explosive temper. She would then try to make it up to me with hugs and kisses.

I loved and resented my mother. But I never doubted her love for me. It was the sun that warmed my days, my shelter in storms.

My father always made me feel unnecessary, a tagalong. It seemed that all his tenderness was taken up by my sister, the first girl after three boys. He appeared to notice me only to reprimand me or to take something away from me.

Young as I was, I sensed my father's integrity. It was at odds with his treatment of me, but it validated my inferiority.

We were raised in a very straightlaced kind of religion. Everything pleasurable was suspect. Hell awaited the poor sinner who dabbled in "joys of the flesh." I knew all about hell, having listened to many a vivid description by shouting evangelists. I knew it was my destination because I was so bad.

Meek, mousy child, how did that heavy conviction of my "badness" enter my heart? Was it because I could never hope to meet the standards set for some impossible angel-child? Or was it because of thoughts I dared not express? Whatever the cause, the guilt, fear, and unworthiness stayed with me.

When did I learn to be an overeater? I was a scrawny child, though we lived on a farm and food was plentiful. I remember looking at a favorite food on my plate and leaving it because I had enough.

As I approached adolescence, we left the farm and moved to town where my father opened a small business. He worked hard but those were Depression years and he didn't have a chance. From plenty of food we fell to scarcity. As a consequence, I grew even thinner and anemic. I had frequent bouts with bronchitis. Is this when I learned to worship food?

I was painfully shy, and though my grades were excellent, I still thought of myself as stupid and bad. After one year at the local college, I boarded a bus with a little cardboard suitcase containing all I owned and headed for the nearest city to find work.

In the year that followed I had seven different jobs. And I fell in love. John was a soldier. We were akin, two people who belonged together. He saw me as beautiful and brave; for him, I began to be what he thought me. I bloomed.

Children of the Depression, we could not afford to marry and have a family. So we waited. I made a bargain with God: We would be "good"—no premarital sex—and God would see that we had a life together.

As U.S. involvement in World War II approached, my fears for John grew. He had been sent to San Francisco for special training. I joined him and we were married. We had two weeks together. Then he was shipped to the Philippines.

I was alone in a strange city, with no friends and a crushing load of anxiety. I began eating. My weight rose to 200 pounds before I knew what was happening. I was appalled. I quickly dieted down to 140 pounds for John's sake. It was not hard.

No sooner had I lost the weight, however, when I became ill. I had fever, nausea, and pain. The doctors could not determine what was wrong. I was hospitalized and put under observation. After two weeks I told them to operate or send me home. They operated and removed a perfectly healthy appendix.

I was doing defense work when the wire came: John was dead. He was captured on Bataan, went through the infamous death march, and died six months later of fever and starvation.

I plunged into a bottomless rage at God. Though I had never regarded Him as loving, I had thought Him just. Now I knew better. In my anger and grief, I shut everyone out. I carried that anger and grief for thirty years.

I do not condemn myself now for the brief period of promiscuity that followed. In my heartbroken loneliness, I looked for something, anything to hold to, even for a little while. When I found myself pregnant, I had no thought of asking help from anyone. I was fiercely determined to keep my baby and give it all my love.

I had been corresponding with a lonely soldier overseas. He was back now, and he wanted to marry me, baby and all. I did not love him, but I accepted him. He needed me, and I needed some kind of life, I thought.

I lost that first baby. Two years later I had two others, little boys, and the realization that I had married an alcoholic.

The "Big Book" of AA speaks of self-interest that places us in a position to be hurt. I knew that our marriage could never be what I hoped for, but I feared that if I left my husband I could not support my children. So I stayed, out of fear and self-interest, and I was in a position to be hurt.

When the youngsters were four and five, we had a third son. Little Johnny was a beautiful, sunny baby, a delight to both of us. But when he was a year old he developed a mysterious illness and after some weeks we had to take him to the hospital where he was given blood transfusions. Then he was sent home, much improved. I sat holding my dear little one on my lap and watched my two older children at play. A feeling of thankfulness welled up in me. For the first time since John's death, I spoke to God: "Thank you for my sons."

Johnny died of leukemia soon afterward. Once again, I closed the door on God. "You've hurt me enough. Let me alone. Forget I'm here."

What did I have left? Two little boys. They became my only reason for existing, and I tried to live my life through them. What a burden I put on them!

My husband's drinking got worse and so did my own disease. My weight climbed past 300 pounds. From time to time I dieted and lost weight. But a terrible craving would begin gnawing at me day and night. Soon, all determination and hope were gone, along with the dieting and the weight loss.

Predictably, the children were not thriving emotionally. Our older son was a quiet, well-behaved boy, very bright in school but withdrawn and unhappy. When he reached puberty, he began to put on excess weight. I watched him become fatter and more detached as he went through high school, but I knew no way to help him. I couldn't help myself.

Our younger child was a fun loving, outgoing boy, a favorite of sorts with his father. But he got into a minor scrape at twelve, and his father never let him forget it. Time after time, my husband drove the boy out of the house at the slightest provocation. Eventually he married and moved away, which relieved some of the strain .

Our older son attended college for one year, during which he made the dean's list. The next year he flunked out due to lack of interest. He got a job working evenings. When he came home he would stay up all night reading, eating, and watching television. He slept all day and got up in time to go to work. That was his life at twenty-four.

I was now fifty-six. I weighed more than 300 pounds. My feet and ankles swelled hugely; I had arthritis in my knees. My blood pressure was at stroke level.

"But my general health is good," I told the doctor.

"You are very sick," said the doctor. "This can kill you. You must lose weight."

I thought it was nice of her to care, but I didn't. Why should I? All I had to look forward to was my husband's retirement in a year, when he would be home all the time, drinking. I had never driven a car, and my husband never took me anywhere. I could not walk a block without becoming winded. I knew that I could never hope for any escape, any pleasure in life except the food with which I sedated myself. My life was over. I was just marking time, waiting for the hearse.

Then one day my obese older son, who had his mother's compulsion, went to an OA meeting. He came home with all the little pamphlets. I observed his enthusiasm with doubt: Would he stay with it or give up after awhile? Loving mother that I am, I figured that if I started this OA thing with my son, it would help him to continue.

So I went to my first meeting. I was wearing my one dress, a homemade cotton print that I had enlarged from the biggest pattern I could find. And I had two front teeth missing; when you weigh 300 pounds, who cares about your teeth?

All I heard that night was weight loss, "get a sponsor" and "keep coming back." It was enough. I got a sponsor, and I kept coming back.

Abstinence was easy. I did not question the why or how, but for the first time I had something that limited my food and, unaccountably, kept me comfortable. I was hungry by mealtime, of course—probably the first real hunger I had felt for years.

I was quite satisfied with this until I began hearing something else at meetings: the Twelve-Step program. I wanted no part of that, thank you. I had no desire for a spiritual life, and as for turning anything over to the likes of the Higher Power I had known—impossible! But they told me that if I did not follow the Steps I would not keep my abstinence. I had tasted hope, and I could not give it up. So I did as I was told as best I could. My recovery began.

Through my shell of bitterness and hopelessness, the therapy of love reached me. Delicate green tendrils took root in the big aching hollow inside me that food could never fill. As my weight dropped, OA friends rejoiced with me.

With gentle but relentless prodding, people called on me to lead meetings, even to speak at other meetings. From the start, I said yes instead of no. I had let fear speak for me long enough; I couldn't live with it any more. Soon the old shyness and fear of people were gone. I was at last free to be myself.

The practicing alcoholic who was my husband now had a new problem. He had been accustomed to a wife who was a doormat, a martyr mother. Without quite knowing what had happened, he found himself confronted by a stranger who said things like, "I think I'll get a wig," and "I'm going to the dentist." The men he worked with razzed him: "She's wearing makeup and getting her hair done? And she stays out late and you don't know where she is? Uh-oh!" Funny they should guess that I was running away from home, one meeting at a time.

Though none of us knew it, my husband was mortally ill. He died a few weeks before he was due to retire. We were able to accept the sad reality of his life and death with compassion: "He loved us as much as he could. He did his best." There was a sense of peace, a release from pain, and that was all.

Abstinence, weight loss, and personal growth do not solve all of life's difficulties. The last two years have been especially trying as I sought solutions to my own and my troubled younger son's problems. But great progress has been made. My older son, for whose sake I came to OA, lost all his excess weight in the first seven months. Now happily married, he has been maintaining the loss for six years.

Throughout the bad times and the good, the love and assistance of OA friends has been there, sustaining me. I am rich in friendship, who once was so destitute. At an age when too many women are living in the past, I am privileged to be growing, learning, sharing in life. Best of all, I am living at peace with God.

In my springtime years I met with disaster: depression, war, and tragic loss. In my summer years I propped up an alcoholic in his sickness and my own. But this is my Indian Summer, my golden autumn. I am glad to be fully alive every day of it.

29

Beyond Affliction

So GREAT HAD BEEN my isolation before coming to OA that not once had I ever told anyone about my bingeing, not even the psychiatrist who treated me for severe depression.

But even in OA it took me a long time to be able to admit that I was a compulsive overeater—even to myself. For nearly one year I remained a "half measure" member, playing around with abstinence, still convinced that my weight was my only problem. I balked at everything from finger salad to God, sure that I was smarter than all that, still in control. And then something unexpected happened that taught me a hard lesson in powerlessness and changed my life.

At the age of twenty-two, almost overnight, I was stricken with a disease that took away ninety percent of my eyesight and left me legally blind, with little hope for any future return of vision. The doctors gave me an apologetic, "There's nothing more we can do," and released me to pursue on my own the channels of state and federal support for the blind.

Understandably, I became despondent and withdrawn. Unfortunately, I also withdrew from OA, which of course led to a resumption of uncontrolled eating. The bingeing progressed in severity, eventually resulting in a violent case of food poisoning. The effect of this illness on my morale was devastating. I hit an emotional bottom lower than I had ever imagined possible.

For a while I thought I was going to die and, indeed, I wondered if that wouldn't be the best solution to my problems. I was so scared and so sick. But lying there that night, trembling and crying, I started to pray—to whom or what I didn't know. Presently, I became aware of something deep within me that didn't want to die, that wanted desperately to live and be free. I continued to pray not to die, to be given another chance.

I know now that this prayer was answered by a God I didn't even believe in at the time, for somehow I found my way back to OA. There, the friends I had made were waiting with open arms and hearts. They took me to meetings, read literature to me, and literally held my hand through days when that was all that would help.

One member had me come and live with her for a while, where she lovingly prepared three abstinent meals each day. Another recorded a Fourth-Step inventory guide on a cassette tape so that I could continue with that important part of the program.

I attended meetings daily and was in the constant company of other OA members. This not only helped keep me abstinent, but it greatly eased the adjustment to my blindness.

But most importantly, as I look back now, I was persuaded, despite my fears, to attend my first OA retreat. There, I received the spiritual counsel from the retreat master to allow myself to feel and acknowledge my grief, and to be honest enough to tell God that I was angry and felt deserted by Him.

This I did with a vengeance, letting out in one afternoon alone in my room years of suppressed hatred for a God I unconsciously blamed for all the unhappiness of my life. To my surprise, when I was through I felt strangely cleansed and relieved of the burden of "God-pleasing" under which I had lived all my life. I had destroyed the fearsome, cruel God of my own making, and was open at last to the discovery of a new God who could be my friend and work with me.

This experience so freed me from the bonds of my physical limitations that I no longer felt oppressed by my blindness, but instead soared in the flight of the spirit. I came to see the difference between my body and my "self," accepting completely my powerlessness over my physical condition. At the same time I accepted responsibility for my spiritual condition: my attitude and the way I live my life.

Although my abstinence had begun on shaky, unsure footing, it grew in strength. As I watched the weeks turn into months and years, I saw my life take on a sanity and serenity I had never known. In addition, a significant percentage of my eyesight returned, and today I am able to work, drive a car, and do almost anything a fully sighted person can do.

It would not be honest to say that the years in OA have been easy. Stripped of the defense of fat (I now maintain a 50-pound weight loss, down from a top weight of 165) and the rationalizations that let me blame everyone else for whatever happened to me, I have had to confront myself head-on. I have had to deal with my many character defects in the slow and arduous process of growing up.

Many times, there have been food problems. Although I have been abstinent from all refined carbohydrates for more than five years now, the pain of an occasional protein binge has knocked me back down to reality and humility: I am a compulsive overeater; I am powerless over food. I am not proud of this particular learning process, nor do I believe it is necessary for others. It just seems to have been the way for me, and that's all I can share.

I have had to learn to accept myself when I fall short, and rather than become despondent over a slip, to pick myself up again and throw myself with confidence and faith all the harder into working my OA program. I cannot count all the times I have called in my food again to a sponsor for a month or so to get myself back on the track. This helps to remind me that I must remain first, last, and always a newcomer in my own mind, and to work my program in that way.

But oh! What treasures I have found through it all. Where once trembled a hurt and frightened little girl now stands a woman with the courage and confidence to live and to love, and to accept what life has to give in return. Through daring to be vulnerable I have been able to form close friendships with many good people, both in and out of OA. And by learning to trust people I have come to trust a God who today is my greatest friend and sponsor, sustaining me through all.

My travels have carried me far, but always I have found the hand of OA stretched out to me. And I in turn have reached out to those who needed me. There is no limit to what can be accomplished in and through the lives of people who partake of the fellowship of Overeaters Anonymous. I know that whatever my future brings, I will be brought again and again into contact with those who can be helped by my experience. And through these contacts, I will be allowed to continue my own progress on this magnificent journey.

30 ⸻

The Valedictorian

IN A FAMILY of painfully thin people, I was labeled the "fat" one. My parents and sisters were so thin they avoided cameras, and the females cried after trying on clothes because they were so bony. During the Depression years it was considered healthy to be plump.

When I look at childhood pictures of myself, I realize that I was quite normal. But I thought of myself as fat.

During adolescence I amazed my friends by eating voraciously without putting on a pound; but by high school graduation I was carrying twenty-five extra pounds, all below the waist, hidden as well as possible by dressing carefully.

The conflict between school and home life was in full bloom. At home I was a clumsy drudge, always striving for perfection (which I thought was possible with a little more effort on my part) and always falling short.

An old French tradition led my parents to seek a balance

in our behavior to avoid that most hateful of sins—conceit. The news of any success at school was met with a reminder of failings at home. My self-esteem was very low, although there were moments of great exhilaration—being valedictorian, winning scholarships, cheerleading, election to organizational offices, and important roles in school plays and as a vocal soloist.

My family thought college was a waste of time for a woman, but allowed me to go when I agreed to pay all costs, provide my own clothing, continue with household chores and make a token payment for room and board. What perverse pride I took in being so self-sufficient! The comfortable feeling of martyrdom took the edge off the hardships. Those were busy years. I was hoping to become a woman lawyer, a rare ambition for a steelworker's daughter in post-World War II days.

I worked in a local dairy store, famous for its imaginative creations at the soda fountain. I began to refer to myself as a "foodaholic." It seemed funny then.

After two years my enthusiasm began to wane when one of my friends became an attorney and related discouraging tales of a woman's limited prospects in that field. It was a period of disenchantment for me. College lost its mystique when the academic work proved easy to master, a pattern that was commonplace in my life.

I frankly felt superior to most of the women I knew and had men pegged as an interesting, if unknown, quantity—but certainly intellectually inferior. The men I would have liked to date were put off by my arrogance.

When I began to date often, my parents were concerned about my sexual behavior. Being supersensitive, I took their inquiries as accusations and determined to rebel in my own way. I soon left school, pregnant, to be married. We had three children and a shaky marriage.

I reveled in my "disgrace." I kept friends and neighbors in stitches, pointing out the short-comings of my husband and my misadventures as a housewife. I used to say that I would rather be hated than pitied. Now I realize that my stories were filled with self-pity and all pointed back to "poor me." I loved to help others but would never accept any help for fear that I would then "owe" someone something.

When I was twenty-eight I learned that I had uterine cancer. I had never heard of anyone who survived such a diagnosis and prepared to face death. I wanted desperately to regain my childhood faith but found it out of my reach. I did survive, more confused than ever. The "spayed dog" jokes began and my weight fluctuated wildly. I became overly protective of my children, who were of school age. It didn't take much encouragement to become the forerunner of today's retread college students, this time as a prospective language teacher.

Eventually I was asked to teach at the university level, a position I loved so much I would have paid to do it. Astonishingly, I was never hungry until I arrived home at night. I could easily fast every day until noon, but the minute I opened the refrigerator all resolve melted. In the past, I had read about celebrities who maintained their figures with creative low-calorie dishes prepared by their cooks. If only I didn't have to spend so much time in the kitchen; if only I didn't have to stretch our budget with high-carbohydrate fillers, I could be slim, too.

I gained another twenty-five pounds which were impossible to hide.

When my youngest son was in high school, I declared my independence from the kitchen and from any valet duties in the house. I stated that we were all adults, that there would be food in the refrigerator, and that each person was responsible for cleaning up after himself.

I was running out of excuses for my overeating. Even declaring my independence from the kitchen didn't stop me.

Then everything fell apart. The industry for which my husband worked closed its doors. He turned increasingly to drink. Times were changing at the university, too. I was publishing but doomed to perish without my Ph.D. My husband started at the bottom in a new job with the merchant marine, and suddenly I was alone and inactive. My weight hit a new high. I was on my way to becoming fat-lady-of-the-circus obese.

It was comforting to stay home because I could see the shock on my friends' faces when I appeared in public. I had always been a chameleon, changing the color of my personality according to what I assumed was my reflected image in the eyes of those around me. I hated that reflection and those who mirrored it. It wasn't the real me!

But maybe it was. The frayed inseams on my pantsuits said so. I was falling down often. What had happened to my figure skater's grace? It came to me that I had chosen one of the ugliest and slowest ways to commit suicide.

After experimenting with every diet plan I read about, I joined a commercial weight-loss group, lost one dress size, and then despaired. I had heard about Alcoholics Anonymous and was jealous that they could attain sobriety while I had to take that first deadly bite to survive.

I saw an article about OA in Dear Abby and sent for information. There was a group in my city. Still, I felt that if I could muster a little self-discipline I could lick the problem. Surely the same drive that had worked so well in school could be channeled into this area.

I had an inspiration. I would make a verbal promise to my husband that when he sailed home again, he would find a thin wife waiting. I could lie to myself, but my word to another was my honor. Oh, how I tried, feeling more hysterical with each failure. My eating was out of control. My hunger was never appeased.

It took me a year to walk into my first OA meeting, humiliated and belligerent. Why should I seek help from a bunch of fatties? (I have since come to love their sensitivity and intelligence.)

"Give me your diet and don't mess with my mind," I told them. They smiled at me. My best sarcasm couldn't penetrate those tolerant smiles. I grabbed some literature. I would read it and judge it and return to tell them how they could improve. Those smiles would evaporate next week.

I lost twenty-six pounds in the first month and it seemed easy. I kept going to meetings, now smiling back at fellow members with silent smugness.

Unfortunately for my plan to sabotage OA, someone lent me a copy of AA's "Big Book." I devoured it in one sitting and began to cry, a feminine weakness I rarely allowed myself. They were telling my story in that book. It took a little translation from alcohol to food, but I recognized myself on every page.

Then my appetite reappeared. I quickly surrendered to it, thinking how little will power it would take to get started again. But I couldn't get restarted, and I learned another truism: It's easier to stay on than to get on.

I went to my next meeting ready to listen to what they were saying about the disease, and it began to make sense—except for some of those Twelve Steps. How could I have injured anyone? Hadn't my veneer of ladylike politeness prevented me from doing anything worse than using witty sarcasm? Later, when writing my Fourth-Step inventory, I was to discover that my frequent expression, "I hate people who . . . and institutions that . . ." was only the tip of an angry, hurtful internal iceberg.

I began to realize that I had been dieting again and that, unless I made some drastic changes in myself, I would never achieve abstinence. I had to stop analyzing and start acting.

Luckily, I was able to attend a state OA convention where a wise speaker told us that our program was a double trail—without working the Step program we would find abstinence impossible, and without abstaining we couldn't work the Step program well. My mind opened just a tiny crack. I had been afraid to be vulnerable, teachable, but with willingness came many good things.

Recently, I visited a friend who was undergoing treatment for alcoholism. "Aren't you afraid that we are being brainwashed?" she asked. We thought about it for a while and came to the mutual conclusion that our whole past had programmed us into negative thinking and that it would take some welcome "brainwashing" to begin to think positively.

My progress has been terribly slow. Being a quick student in school hadn't helped my plan of action. Often, those whom I sponsor seem to take gigantic leaps forward, inspiring me instead of vice versa. After two and a half years, I have finally lost all but ten pounds of my excess weight, and I have maintained instead of gaining during the plateaus.

My family life has become a great joy to me. What a reve-lation to find that my husband manages his life much better alone than when it was a joint venture. I simply had to step back to appreciate what he is—a much better person than I was trying to make of him.

My children willingly communicate now without having to defend every action. When I talk with my mother, I know that she has a right to her own actions and that my only responsibility is to love her and control my reactions. Before, the slightest hesitation in her voice told me I had displeased her and threw me into a panic.

I no longer see myself and my world as a reflection in the eyes of others. My perceptions come from a new confidence in my ability to view my surroundings without judgment.

A day of abstinence in my life is a thing of beauty. The fattest abstinent person at a meeting is in a better place than I am if I don't have abstinence.

I have become aware that I have an addictive personality. Maybe that's why I unconsciously denied myself too much liquor, too much impulsive spending.

I find that the void left by all these potential addictions is being filled by the only healthy addiction I have—love. I accept that there is a power greater than myself and that the love that flows from it enables me to stand ready to love every person with whom I have contact—even the one in the mirror.

It's funny how nice other people have become. On my last birthday I welcomed being forty-eight because physically, spiritually, and emotionally I am a much better me than I have ever been.

Someone told me that I have a long way to go if I expect

the world to be equitable and fair. I'll never be well, but I am getting better. I have fallen on my face dozens of times, but I can stop branding myself a failure and, with the direction of my Higher Power, pick myself up and grow—a day at a time.

31 ———

Compulsive Like Me

I WAS ONE OF six children. My family, of Italian extraction, started out well but the Depression touched our lives as it did so many.

I can remember some very happy times but I also remember never having enough of anything, not even necessities such as food and clothing. Though I was not fat as a child, I could never get my fill of food. Whenever I could, I stole pennies and bought candy or cookies. When my father became ill we moved from the city to a small community near the ocean. Our new house was built on stilts and stood at the end of a street that backed up to a canal. The canal became a means of survival for the family. We fished, rented rowboats, and sold fish door to door. We ate fish two or three times a day. Fried eels was not an unusual breakfast.

Parental discipline was so strict that even as a teenager I was not allowed to date or wear makeup. As I began to earn money, I bought junk food and filled up on it before going home to a pot of whatever my mother had cooked, mostly starches. This practice launched me on what I knew was a very selfish, sneaky way to live.

At sixteen, I was five-foot, one-inch tall and a dumpy 128 pounds. When one of my sisters made fun of me, I went on a dill pickle diet to lose weight. I lost the weight, but I became run down and caught a cold that turned into a severe case of pneumonia.

In the hospital I was so close to death, a priest gave me final rites. In the worst stage of my illness I kept asking for the man I was to marry, whom I had met and fallen in love with when I was fourteen. He came to my bedside with his sister and gave me a friendship ring. I started a great recovery. We dated after that, but only on Sundays, and I had to be home at ten, a curfew my father imposed.

Father was a wine alcoholic, and he was usually drunk. Every week he embarrassed me and tormented my mother trying to get her to promise that she would take me for a Monday morning checkup to see if I was still a virgin. She never did. I was twenty years old and a virgin when I was married.

In the next two years, through pregnancy and pounds gained and lost, I tried unsuccessfully to get down to my normal size. There was no doubt now about my compulsion to overeat. One day, fat and unhappy at 130 pounds, I happened to read a book about the Roman Empire. It told of feasts lasting several days and the beautiful marble basins called vomitoriums where wealthy Romans and their guests induced vomiting in order to be able to continue eating and drinking.

The ugly seed was planted. Not long after reading that book I bought a huge strawberry shortcake. I sat down with a cup of coffee and ate one piece after another until I had finished the cake. Nausea swept over me. I barely made it to the bathroom where the whole cake came up. It was unpleasant, but afterward I felt good. A few days later I repeated the performance.

I regarded this incredible feat as my own secret discovery. It was as though I had a special trick, and whenever I felt like eating some food that took my fancy, I performed this trick. The weight fell off. At 110 pounds I felt very comfortable. Now, how does an overeater stay at 110? By eating and throwing up. I did it for nearly thirty years. My wardrobe size never changed. My family and friends marveled at the food I could consume without getting fat. They said, "Isn't she lucky, she can eat anything and everything and not gain a pound." I heard remarks like that all my adult life, and I cringed with guilt.

But I had become an accomplished sneak and conniver. Years went by and slim, trim Cora remained the same. At first I binged every couple of months, then monthly, weekly, daily and finally three or four times a day. I couldn't understand why I did it. Each day I made a solemn vow to stop. I must never put my fingers down my throat again, I told myself. But I couldn't stop. I wanted more and more food. Huge quantities of all sorts of food. It got to a point where I didn't choose anything. It just became everything in sight.

My ritual was always the same: I would eat until my stomach hurt. I had to stand very straight in order not to feel the terrible discomfort. Then I would run to the bathroom and turn on the tap so no one would hear me. I always washed my hands because I didn't want a disease in my mouth. The disease that was in my head raged unchecked.

Years passed, and I saw my own daughter and my sisters getting fat. Many times it occurred to me to tell them my secret, but I was ashamed. In thirty years I never broke my silence.

When my sister began attending OA meetings, she sent literature about the program to my daughter who by now weighed more than 200 pounds. I had been praying for her, not yet aware of how sick I was. But I was close to the bottom of the pit. I wanted to stop. Each time I looked into the toilet bowl, fear gripped me. I thought, someday I am going to die right here locked in the bathroom. Alone.

One day, I could not vomit. The muscles in my throat refused to work. I kept trying, defiant and full of fear at the same time.

"Oh my God," I thought. "I've done it. I ruined my throat." The next day I was so nervous and afraid, I didn't eat. My dilemma was indescribable.

At this point my daughter, who was now in OA, opened a door that was to show me the way out. She invited me to go to a meeting so I could meet her friends. I went and I listened. I bought some literature, and I started my secret OA. I cold-turkeyed alone. How could I ask anyone to sponsor me? Overeaters were fat; I was thin.

I took God as my sponsor. Each day I said the Serenity Prayer. I did not know how much I could eat and not gain weight. But I had stopped putting my fingers down my throat. Joyfully, through this program and God's grace, I have just celebrated four years of freedom from that obsession.

After one and a half years of working the program alone, I was still afraid. My weight was slowly creeping up. I reached 124 pounds. Here was another turning point, a new decision to be faced: throw up or get fat—or come out of the closet.

I chose to live. I chose OA. I humbled myself and walked into a room full of overweight people. They stared at me. But I needed them. I took a sponsor and began abstinence, which I have had one day at a time for the past two and a half years.

What a joy to get on the scale once a week and find my weight 107 or 108 pounds! It has been a beautiful four years. At first, weight loss was my goal. After reaching it I chose two new goals. One is to grow emotionally and the other, spiritually. It hasn't been an easy road. After years of giving my life nothing but guilt, misery, fear, depression, and no self-worth, I have had restored to me the soundness of mind and body that was God's gift to me at birth.

How blessed I feel that the people in OA didn't judge me as different but understood that I have the same food compulsion they have. Their acceptance opened the doors to so much for me. I have learned how to be honest. My first amends were to my daughter. I told her everything, and from that moment on I felt I wasn't alone anymore. It embarrasses her to hear that she saved my life, but it's true.

Finally, I told my husband. I had been hiding literature and going to meetings secretly. He was shocked. But I went on to ask his pardon for all the food money I stole and for the lavish meals I let him buy me only to feed my obsession.

Now I have a new peace. I had been a human ship, tossing about in life, looking for a port—and at last I found one.

OA is my resting place, my comfort, my serenity, and joy. I shall never, and can never, go back to that stormy sea of food obsession.

Appendices

A Disease of the Mind

Several years ago, as a psychiatrist working in drug abuse and alcoholism programs, I was led through the experience of a staff member to examine compulsive overeating as a disease process identical to alcoholism. We started to apply, in a limited fashion, the same principles to the problem of compulsive overeating that we were using in our alcoholism treatment program, and found them to be very successful. The more closely I examined the phenomenon, the clearer it became that compulsive overeating is a disease.

In medical school, we doctors are never taught about overeating, certainly not as a disease. So we are prejudiced against it. Overeaters Anonymous is very successful with cases that haven't responded to conventional kinds of treatment. This success is often threatening to the professionals because it's difficult for us to see how someone who hasn't had years of study and experience could be more successful with people we've been trying to treat, unsuccessfully, for so long.

The remarkable thing about OA's success is that the program gets people to function far better than they ever have in their lives. With any other disease, you're lucky to get back to where you were. If you have a heart attack, for example, you're fortunate to get your heart to function as well as it did before the attack.

With the compulsive overeater, not only do you get back to a normal weight but, more importantly, your life is changed and in a sense you're ahead of where you were before you became a compulsive overeater. Now you have tools of feeling, touching, caring, loving, sharing, being honest with your family, and looking at life in an understanding way and not fighting it but going along with it. Once you treat the illness, you have the potential for a more "together" person than you were. Therefore, it's exciting for physicians and others who have been ignoring the problem or expressing deep pessimism about it, to think of compulsive overeating as a disease and to realize that it can be treated so successfully.

One of the prejudices about compulsive overeating is society's view of a compulsive overeater as someone who is obese. Yet the overeater can be one pound overweight or even underweight, as in anorexia nervosa, and still be a compulsive overeater. The illness has nothing to do with weight. That's why it's so silly to go on diets or to weigh oneself all the time.

The problem is with the control of food. Is one preoccupied with controlling food intake to the point that it's interfering with one's life? Just as being an alcoholic is not related to the amount one drinks, being a compulsive overeater is not related to the amount one weighs.

The overeater's problem is not being able to control eating behavior the way other people can, and the need is for a system to control that behavior. Of course, the most effective one is a support system like that of Overeaters Anonymous. What the overeater has to do is turn over the control to a Higher Power. Once it is turned over, the behavior is under control.

A major confusion we in medicine have is the erroneous belief that compulsive overeating is a result of physiologic, psychologic, and environmental problems. We try to treat compulsive overeaters psychiatrically or physically with medicine or structures in their lives, and it doesn't work. The reason it fails is because we are doing it in reverse. What has to be dealt with is the compulsive overeating. When it is, the physiologic and psychiatric problems seem to take care of themselves.

There are some people, about the same percentage as in the general population, who, after getting the food back in its proper place, find themselves needing traditional psychiatric care because they do have a problem which they pushed down with food. But that is the exception. What is probably true in most cases is that the individual develops the compulsive overeating mechanism for dealing with life at an early age and then starts to push problems down with the food. Once people become compulsive overeaters, every aspect of their lives is affected. Now they get into the psychological, physical, and environmental problems and start changing their lives, their friends, and their social structure. All these changes are really caused by the compulsive overeating. Most compulsive overeaters, through a program like OA's, will lose all these syndromes and not need to have any kind of traditional psychiatric care.

We in the medical community must take responsibility for failing to understand the real problem. Compulsive overeating is a serious disease, and it is devastating this country. It is the basic cause of disorders which medicine views as primary illnesses, such as hypertension and diabetes. But physicians don't look at compulsive overeating, they look at the secondary disease process which comes from compulsive overeating. They ignore the overeating and rigorously work on the symptoms and the secondary diseases.

Obviously, that is not the way to treat it. If a patient has pneumonia, the doctor doesn't treat the fever and then send the patient home after the temperature is normal, saying "Your fever is down; now watch that pneumonia." But we certainly do this with the overeater. We take care of the symptoms of the secondary disease and we tell that patient, "Your weight (or blood pressure, or blood sugar) is normal; now watch that overeating."

It is the responsibility of the medical community to understand what compulsive overeating really means and to recognize that Overeaters Anonymous has been dealing successfully with the disease. We need to work closely with OA, to have OA as the base or structure, and only then should we offer what we as professionals are able to contribute. The doctor should have the patient go to OA, and then serve as OA's support system for that patient. Overeaters Anonymous should be the treatment and the professional should be the adjunct, not the other way around. This is very difficult for a physician or mental health professional to accept.

As long as Overeaters Anonymous continues to keep the principles it has now, it will be our most valuable means of treatment of the disease of compulsive overeating. OA's principles ensure that no individual has power. In essence, it is a leaderless organization, making the process much stronger than any one member or group.

Overeaters Anonymous is a system of people who are trying to help each other, and as such it is tremendously successful.

William Rader, M.D.

Dr. Rader is a psychiatrist engaged in clinical work with alcohol, drug addiction and compulsive overeating. Winner of the 1977 Appreciation Award of Overeaters Anonymous, he has carried the OA message both in his treatment programs and in a number of local and national television documentaries. He is currently chairman of the board for MEDRA, a multinational program for the advancement of alternative medicine.

A Disease of the Body

I was most pleased, several years ago, to be invited as a representative of the American Society of Bariatric Physicians (a medical scientific society devoted to the study of obesity and allied conditions) to attend an annual convention of Overeaters Anonymous. I have since then attended several others. I was also privileged to attend some local group meetings.

The basic concept of Overeaters Anonymous is that compulsive overeating is a disease which affects the person on three levels—physical, spiritual, and emotional. Members of OA feel that, like alcoholics, they are unable to control their compulsion permanently by unaided will power.

Obesity is unquestionably one of the major health problems in the United States today. In fact, it is a problem common to all affluent societies. Estimates as to the number of overweight individuals in the United States range from ten million to more than seventy million, depending on what criteria are used to classify an individual as obese. Furthermore, in recent years there has been a steady increase in the number of overweight individuals. This is due to many factors. Chief among them is our success in creating an abundant food supply while our physical activity continues to diminish.

To indicate the magnitude of this menace, a Gallup Poll in 1973 revealed that 46 percent of Americans polled felt they were overweight, while less than 8 percent thought they were underweight. Out of every ten persons, four or five were doing something to control their weight. Senator George McGovern's committee hearings disclosed that obesity nourishes a ten-billion-dollar industry, with 100 million dollars yearly being spent for reducing drugs alone. The US.Public Health Service estimates that at least 60 million Americans weigh more than they should. The most disturbing problem is that perhaps less than five percent of dieters are able to maintain weight loss for at least five years.*

As a physician, my main concern with the obese is the medical risks to which their obesity exposes them. Such per-

---

*As of 2000, 55 percent, or 97 million adults, in the US are overweight or obese, with at least 33 percent of adults considered overweight and 22 percent considered obese. Obesity-related medical conditions now contribute to 300,000 deaths in the US each year. The total US costs attributable to obesity amounted to over $99 billion in 1995; over half of those dollars were direct medical costs. Obesity has been recognized since 1985 as a chronic disease and is now the second leading cause of preventable death, exceeded only by cigarette smoking. (http://www.asbp.org/bariatrics)

sons have a greater than 40 percent chance of dying in any given year from heart disease, a greater than 30 percent chance of dying from coronary artery disease, a greater than 50 percent death rate from cerebrovascular disease (strokes) as well as an increased death rate from many other diseases. It has also been pointed out recently that the risk of developing diabetes is increased two-fold by an increase of 20 percent in body weight. In women, there is also a significant increase in the development of uterine cancer associated with excess body weight. In a recent study of 75,532 fat women, there were sixteen diseases associated with obesity. Furthermore, obesity predisposes to high blood pressure, gallbladder disease and the formation of gallstones requiring surgery. Even babies born of obese mothers have more than twice the infant mortality of babies whose mothers' weights are normal.

Most individuals who join Overeaters Anonymous are aware of these risks. But, like alcoholics, they are unable to control their compulsion on any lasting basis. They have completely lost faith in life and in themselves. In OA, the hand of understanding and strength is extended to them by people who suffer the same compulsion and who are now examples that there is an answer. This probably explains OA's success with the hopeless obese person who has repeatedly failed with the usual methods of weight control. I was particularly impressed with the extreme friendliness and even love between members that was easily observable at meetings.

Many OA members are former participants (and dropouts) of commercial weight control groups. I observed a number of individuals who had been unsuccessful in the commercial organizations, but who had reached and maintained normal weight for a number of years after having joined Overeaters Anonymous. On being asked why they switched organizations, they were quick to inform me that the continual preparation of "free" foods and general preoccupation with food, as sometimes expounded, only kept their food compulsion alive.

When compulsive overeaters realize that they cannot control their eating behavior, they need to accept and depend upon another power—a power acknowledged to be greater than oneself. The interpretation of this power is left to the individual. Many, perhaps most, members of OA adopt the concept of God. But newcomers are merely asked to keep an open mind on this subject and usually they find it is not too difficult to work out a solution to this very personal problem, even if they are atheist or agnostic.

Psychologically, the obese individual is helped to attain a sense of the reality and nearness of a greater power which replaces one's egocentric nature. Then the person's point of view and outlook will take on a spiritual coloring. Hence, one no longer needs to maintain a defiant individuality but can live in peace and harmony with the environment, sharing and participating freely, especially with other members of the group. This is a great therapeutic weapon that I, as a physician who has dealt with obese people for more than twenty-seven years, can appreciate. The obese individual no longer defies, but accepts help, guidance, and control from the outside. As OA members relinquish their negative, aggressive feelings toward themselves and toward life, they find themselves overwhelmed by positive feelings of love, friendliness, tranquility, and a pervading contentment.

These latter feelings were evident among the groups I attended.

A word frequently heard in OA groups is surrender. It can best be described as letting go. The individual gives up personal rigidities, relaxes and admits to being beaten by compulsive overeating. The source of this feeling is almost always despair, which is so prevalent in newcomers to the group. It is all part of a crisis experience with an overload of hopelessness. In the act of surrender, one does not just give up but accepts a power greater than oneself, reducing the ego and admitting the need for outside help.

The "ego reduction" can be very profitable to the personality makeup of this person. It is important to differentiate between submission and surrender. In submission, an individual accepts reality consciously, but not unconsciously. There is acceptance that one cannot, at the moment, conquer reality, but lurking in the unconscious is the feeling that "there will come a day when I will be able to handle my problem on my own."

Submission implies no real acceptance of one's inadequacy; on the contrary, it demonstrates conclusively that the struggle is still going on. Submission is, at best, a superficial yielding, with the inner tensions still present. When the individual accepts, on an unconscious level, the reality of not being able to handle compulsive overeating, there is no residual battle. Relaxation ensues with a freedom from strain and conflict. This freedom is the aim of the OA groups, and complete surrender is manifested by the considerable degree of relaxation which is evident in the behavior of those who have achieved it.

Once compulsive overeaters surrender at the unconscious level, their compliance with the disciplines of the program does not lessen with time, leading to the inevitable regaining of weight. They continue to get messages from the unconscious that the need for outside help will remain for a prolonged, if not indefinite period. Their wholehearted cooperation is then forthcoming, and constructive action takes the place of skin-deep assurances that they will merely comply temporarily until the memory of their suffering and self-pity weakens and the need for compliance lessens.

Surrender, then, is an unconscious event. It is not willed by the individual. It can occur only when one becomes involved with one's unconscious mind in a set of circumstances which signal the undeniable need for an external greater power. The definition of surrender can be understood only when all its unconscious ramifications and true inner meaning are glimpsed. Observed by others, such an individual manifests an inner calm and a "live and let live" attitude.

In analyzing Overeaters Anonymous, I have reached a number of conclusions. There appears to be a deep shift in the individual's emotional tone, the disappearance of one set of feelings, and the emergence of a very different set. The member moves from a negative state of mind to a positive one. This may have the earmarks of a spiritual conversion. Be that as it may, it is an effective transformation and essential for long-term success.

By this I do not mean to imply that there are never any slipups. Indeed, there are. But they are usually due to overconfidence as people are successful in the program and once again become too preoccupied with themselves. As long as they attend group meetings, help is immediately available, inspiring them to return to abstinence and to the Twelve Steps of recovery. They are neither judged nor scolded. There are no weigh-ins. They can share their past experiences, their present problems and their hopes for the future with those who understand and support them and who speak their own language. Working with a sponsor, the individual converses with a person who has been through similar experiences. Thus the communication between these two is on the same level. When OAers become sponsors themselves, their loneliness is greatly alleviated. They are needed and accepted. This has a very potent, positive influence on weight maintenance.

OA literature suggests that the newcomer visit a doctor to decide upon a plan of eating suited to both physical needs and family habits. I can verify that this was, indeed, the policy with a number of patients whom I have referred to this group. OA is not concerned with the medical aspects of obesity, but with the compulsive nature of overeating.

It is my firm belief that Overeaters Anonymous has made a definite place for itself in helping the obese individual and renders a valuable service to such a person. The empathy and attention individuals receive at meetings during trying times can be of great therapeutic value. Overeaters Anonymous can help individuals restore their faith in themselves and in others and give them hope for recovery. There is no other organization, lay or professional, that has such a profound influence on the compulsive overeater's thinking; and, after all, it is our thoughts that precede our emotions, and it is our emotions that make us eat inappropriately and become physically obese. Recovery in OA is on all three levels. It may seem a tall order, but one which has the greatest chance for success.

It has been an honor and a most exciting experience for me as a professional to have had the opportunity to get to know the members of Overeaters Anonymous. I will forever be grateful to them for the good work they do in combating a major health problem in the United States.

Peter G. Lindner, M.D.

Dr. Lindner was past president of the American Society of Bariatric Physicians and chairman of its board of trustees. He received the 1975 Appreciation Award of Overeaters Anonymous in recognition of his work in the field of obesity and compulsive overeating and his efforts to bring the OA program to the attention of the medical community and the general public. Dr. Lindner passed away in 1987.

APPENDIX **C**

A Disease of the Spirit

The title of this commentary puts in simple words the uniqueness and special place that Overeaters Anonymous has earned and is earning within the whole approach to the problem of compulsive overeating.

It was not easy to determine how to apply a program dealing with alcoholism, in which thousands have learned how to live without drinking, to a commodity—food—without which not one can live. I am sure that this difficulty still exists within the minds of some. For many others, however, it is clear that what compulsive overeaters and alcoholics have in common is a need to nourish the spiritual side of their nature.

All in all, it is the saving grace of the spiritual in the OA program that has made for its success and growth, and I can prophesy that OA will continue to grow, bringing not only sane eating habits, but spiritually and morally oriented lives that will help build society.

Spiritual values are important because they deal with the whole person. Wholeness in this sense is related to "holiness," as well as to "balance." A holy person is one whose body, mind, and spirit share an equality that was (and is) the intention and plan of God for all men. Such a person takes his or her place within the community with ease and grace, motivated by a deep and abiding sense of thanksgiving. Such individuals become creative and constructive, not only with the family circle or community but in the arts and sciences. Their creative energies are not blocked by shame, guilt, self-pity, and hate, nor by the facades of arrogance, aggressiveness, and uncaring attitudes.

It is only as the hurt and damaged soul is given emotional and spiritual sustenance that these destructive characteristics slough off, and love begins to flow freely within and from there outward.

Let us look at this spiritual food. To begin with, it falls under the heading of love, the most abused, misused, and yet the most wonderful word in the English language. Without love, every other human virtue or ability is as "sounding brass." Love is a spiritual quality that is not confined to the limits of any religious community. No one has a corner on it. It is free—free to fill the lives of all who allow it to flow freely. And as it flows, it both washes and gives life and glorifies its source—God.

This brings me to my first point. Those who are prone to stuff themselves with food that makes their bodies unsightly are refusing the food that satisfies and soothes the unhappy soul within. Have they said, "I don't deserve anything good" for such a long time that they are literally putting their heels on that source of love that alone can bring peace? Or have they become so discouraged or so angry that they deny even the existence of love, let alone God?

All of us can identify with such feelings. Compulsive overeaters and alcoholics, gamblers and drug addicts are not the only inhabitants of life's gray areas. The number of such afflicted people is legion.

There are three stages in the process of getting any kind of food. One: Take your body to the food. Two: Dish it out and eat it. Three: Enjoy it and use the energy it creates. It is the same with spiritual food, food for the soul. Let us look at these three stages.

One: Take your body to the food. Sometimes people become so sick with overeating that the "spiritual food" has to come through one who cares, one who loves. This is God's method. He first loved us. But sometimes He knocks at the door of our lives in the form of a person or a book or magazine article—a thought, a hope.

The knocking is heard but often the door remains shut. Sooner or later, however, it must be opened to allow some kind of help to enter. In most cases, many kinds of "help" have been tried. They all involved money, effort, and disappointment. Finally, the message gets through: Someone cared enough to reach the starving soul. You allow love within your life. You are ready to take your body to spiritual food.

Two: This stage follows closely upon the accomplishment of the first. How surprising to find—and difficult to believe— that all those people at the OA meeting understood your problem and cared about you !

You see, love that is accepted immediately eliminates your aloneness. The only way you can use the word love when you are alone is by loving yourself, and no compulsive overeater does that at first. So it must begin by allowing someone else's love into your life. This very action of including others and being included is food for the soul—the starving waif within the stuffed body.

But the process of love has only begun. Carefully, even suspiciously, you allow a few people closer to your inner self. Through trusting them, even passively, you move closer to love. You may call these individuals foolhardy to love you, but the pain and loneliness drive you to respond. It becomes easier and easier, until you "over-love" and someone lets you down. This happens because immature love tries to possess and control. Then, you may run back into your shell to lick your wounds, and perhaps a few platters in the process. Like a mighty flood, you feel swamped again by that compulsion that once all but destroyed your life. A phone call: an understanding member of OA hears your story and levels with you. Thankfully, there are many who have learned the difference between loving and "over-loving." They are always standing by, ready to help.

What a relief to be on the raft of OA again—that group of people who take you firmly by the hand in love and fellowship.

It is then that you are encouraged to ingest and digest two new kinds of food: First, understanding for your straightjacketed mind. This comes from OA literature and other sources. Secondly, you learn that prayer and meditation have a lot to do with satisfying the inner hungry one. Finally, you can listen to the stories you hear at meetings with a deeper insight. You study the Traditions, born out of pain and trial, which have kept a spiritual movement living and growing for nearly seventy years. You learn that others have personal histories more traumatic than yours. You acquire humility. You learn some of the tricks of the trade of wholesome living. And finally you can turn to the healthy sauce of good humor. You can not only laugh at the ridiculous reasoning and situations others go through, but you learn to laugh at yourself.

Humor is a most important ingredient of love. I think it shakes down the food—now shrinking away—so that you can make room within yourself for others. This is a major step forward because it takes some of the emotional heat (condemnation) off yourself. And what a relief this is!

Fellowship, understanding, and humor—all of them digestible forms of love: food for the soul.

Somewhere along this pathway the spiritual itself becomes real to you. You begin to be aware of mystical qualities that become important and real. Is this the birth of a soul? No, because the soul was not dead. It was only starving, denied, and stifled. Now it moves within, purring with contentment as it begins its lifelong, God-given task of furnishing control, establishing security and, finally, giving purpose. Now you understand what it was that really attracted you to Overeaters Anonymous. Sure, you were impressed by a slim and trim figure. You wanted that, too. But what really caught you was the love, the understanding, the soul qualities that touched you where you really lived, though you may not have been aware of it.

And wonder of wonders, you too become an instrument of love. You doubted that you could meet the needs of others, but soon the people about you began to respond to your love. Now, you have reached the third stage. You are walking on Cloud Nine, only to be tripped up by pride and even a tinge of complacency or arrogance. The power you envied in others is now yours. You must learn to use it without losing your way again.

Sometimes this experience strands us on a stagnant, arid plateau. You may see someone else maturing more rapidly than you. Disillusionment and standstill can result. There is at this crossroads a signpost you cannot miss: "Go deeper with others and with God."

God has provided many other means of fellowship and growth. They too offer soul-food. But always remember that your compulsion with food does demand that kind of understanding and experience that members of OA can provide. But now that your body is no longer your master; your mind is beginning to think clearly; and your soul is fed, nurtured, and functioning, you can reconsider those other sources of soul food.

I now leave off my description of this pilgrim's progress which takes us from compulsive overeating to its replacement with food for the soul. It is a journey that leads straight out of self-made prisons and limitations into green pastures where we find many a table spread with wholesome food and a cup that overflows.

The Reverend Rollo M. Boas

One of OA's earliest supporters, Rev. Boas was a minister of the Episcopal church and the recipient of OA's 1979 Appreciation Award. He passed away in 1993.

The Twelve Traditions

1. Our common welfare should come first; personal recovery depends upon OA unity.

2. For our group purpose there is but one ultimate authority—a loving God as He may express Himself in our group conscience. Our leaders are but trusted servants; they do not govern.

3. The only requirement for OA membership is a desire to stop eating compulsively.

4. Each group should be autonomous except in matters affecting other groups or OA as a whole.

5. Each group has but one primary purpose—to carry its message to the compulsive overeater who still suffers.

6. An OA group ought never endorse, finance, or lend the OA name to any related facility or outside enterprise, lest problems of money, property, and prestige divert us from our primary purpose.

7. Every OA group ought to be fully self-supporting, declining outside contributions.

8. Overeaters Anonymous should remain forever non-professional, but our service centers may employ special workers.

9. OA, as such, ought never be organized; but we may create service boards or committees directly responsible to those they serve.

10. Overeaters Anonymous has no opinion on outside issues; hence the OA name ought never be drawn into public controversy.

11. Our public relations policy is based on attraction rather than promotion; we need always maintain personal anonymity at the level of press, radio, films, television, and other public media of communication.

12. Anonymity is the spiritual foundation of all these Traditions, ever reminding us to place principles before personalities.

Permission to use the Twelve Traditions of Alcoholics Anonymous for adaptation granted by AA World Services, Inc.

APPENDIX E

To Find Overeaters Anonymous

You can find OA in most cities across the United States and in over fifty-two countries worldwide. Most groups maintain telephone directory listings under "Overeaters Anonymous."

Many groups also place announcements giving a local telephone contact number in the community listings or in the classified section of newspapers.

If there are no public listings of OA groups in your area, or if you need information about OA in other countries, write or call the World Service Office, PO Box 44020, Rio Rancho, NM 87174-4020 USA, 505-891-2664, or check the Web site at: www.overeatersanonymous.org

The international headquarters for Overeaters Anonymous, the World Service Office, maintains up-to-date meeting directories, publishes OA literature, and provides a broad range of other services for groups, intergroups, national and language service boards, and regional offices throughout the world.

OA Publications

Books

The Twelve Steps and Twelve Traditions of Overeaters Anonymous
The Twelve-Step Workbook
For Today
Beyond Our Wildest Dreams
Lifeline Sampler
Abstinence
A New Beginning: Stories of Recovery from Relapse
Voices of Recovery
Seeking the Spiritual Path

Periodical

Lifeline magazine

The World Service Office has over 100 literature items to support
you in your program. Contact the World Service Office
for a catalog of available OA materials.
You may also order material online at
www.oa.org

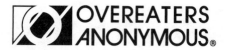